GI
Basics

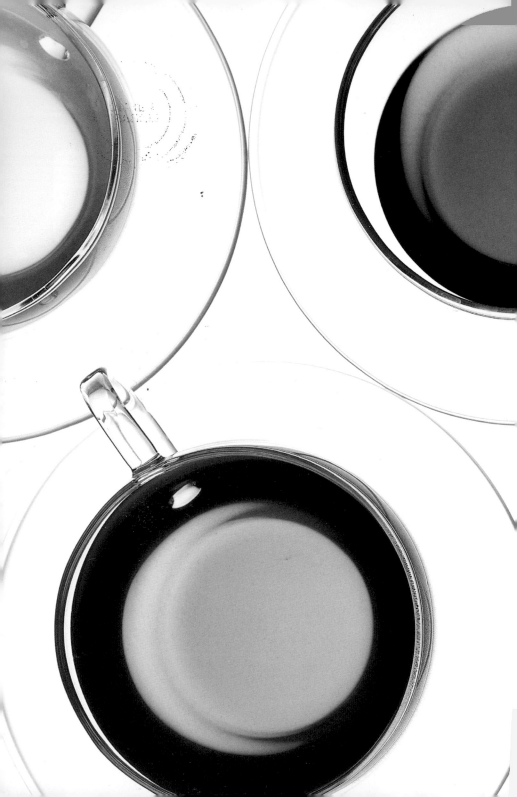

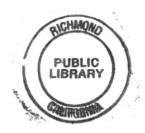

GI
Basics

The low glycemic way to lose weight
and gain energy

Helen Foster

hamlyn

A Pyramid Paperback

First published in Great Britain in 2006 by
Hamlyn, a division of Octopus Publishing Group Ltd
2–4 Heron Quays, London E14 4JP

Copyright © Octopus Publishing Group Limited 2006

Distributed in the United States and Canada by
Sterling Publishing Co., Inc.
387 Park Avenue South, New York, NY 10016-8810

This material was previously published as *Easy GI Diet*

ISBN-13: 978-0-600-61505-7

ISBN-10: 0-600-61505-7

A CIP catalogue record for this book is available from the British Library

Printed and bound in China

10 9 8 7 6 5 4 3 2 1

GI Basics is meant to be used as a general reference and recipe book to aid weight loss. However, you are urged
to consult a health-care professional to check whether it is a suitable weight loss plan for you, before
embarking on it.

While all reasonable care has been taken during the preparation of this edition, neither the publishers, editors,
nor the author can accept responsibility for any consequences arising from the use of this information.

NOTES
This books includes dishes made with nuts and nut derivatives. It is advisable for those with known allergic
reactions to nuts and nut derivatives and those who may be potentially vulnerable to these allergies, such as
pregnant and nursing mothers, invalids, the elderly, babies, and children, to avoid dishes made with nuts and nut
oils. It is also prudent to check the labels of preprepared ingredients for the possible inclusion of nut derivatives.

Meat and poultry should be cooked thoroughly. To test if poultry is cooked, pierce the flesh through the thickest
part with a skewer or fork—the juices should run clear, never pink or red.

All the recipes in this book have been analyzed by a professional nutritionist. The analysis refers to each serving.

Contents

Introduction

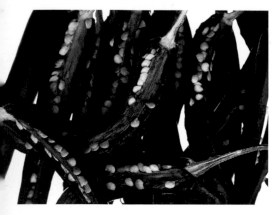

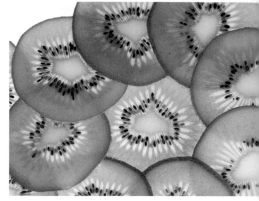

What did you eat today? Does toast and juice for breakfast, a sandwich for lunch, and a bowl of pasta for dinner sound familiar? It probably does, as it is the staple diet of so many of us. Most people would think it was also a pretty healthy diet, as it is low in fat and high in energy-giving carbohydrates. It will therefore surprise you to discover that by eating such a diet you could be increasing your risk of heart problems, diabetes, weight gain, and possibly even some cancers. The truth is that everything we have learned about nutrition over the years is currently being turned on its head.

Too much of a good thing

Back in our grandparents' day, the average person ate 10–13 different types of food a day; today the average person eats 6–8. And the majority of these foods come from one main food group—carbohydrates, and primarily white bread, potatoes, cakes, cookies, and sugary treats. While they may taste good and be easy to eat, these foods create reactions in our bodies that put the entire system out of balance. This is bad news as balance is what our entire system craves—scientists call it homeostasis. The result of imbalance is day-to-day problems such as fatigue, mood swings, and sugar cravings—plus an increased risk of a number of different health problems in the future.

This may not sound new to you. After all, high-protein diets are now very popular, and in these diets carbohydrates are severely

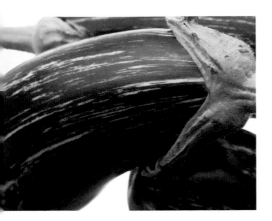
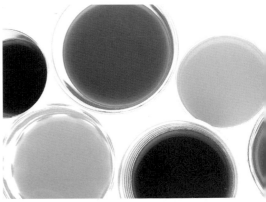

restricted or even banned entirely. And while it's true that these plans help us overcome the side effects of carbohydrate overload, they can bring with them problems of their own such as bad breath, digestive disorders, and overworked kidneys. The results are no less confusing to our systems than what's gone before. There is, however, a better way to eat which stops all the confusion and allows your body to develop a sense of balance without any harmful side effects. It is based on what scientists call the glycemic index, or GI.

A new way of eating

Put very simply, the glycemic index measures how the food you eat reacts in your body. By following a low-GI diet, you choose foods that create only a positive reaction. It sounds simple—and it is. So simple, in fact, that nutritionists are hailing GI as the buzzword for eating in the 21st century, and researchers at the prestigious Harvard University in the USA are producing guidelines based around a low-GI diet which they hope will soon become the national blueprint for health. Forward-thinking countries like Australia are actually marking food packaging with a GI rating to help consumers make the right choice. Eating a low-GI diet is the ultimate way forward when it comes to boosting your health.

GI explained

This chapter will clearly explain exactly what the glycemic index is all about and why it has so many positive effects in your body.

You will discover all the health-boosting benefits that a low-GI diet can bring, everything from reducing your risk of heart disease to cutting your chance of developing wrinkles.

Finally, in this section you will be able to take a quick and easy test to show how your current diet compares, giving you a great baseline to work from when it comes to improving your diet, your body, and your mind.

What is GI?

Every day your body has to take over 10,000 steps, think 40,000 thoughts, pump 8,000 gallons of blood round your system, and deal with all the stresses and strains of modern life. To do this it needs energy—and it gets that energy from food.

The secret of glucose and the glycemic index

The body's preferred fuel is a sugar called glucose, which it makes from starches and sugars (carbohydrates) found in the food that we eat. Glucose is made in the liver after the food has been digested in the stomach.

The converted glucose is then sent to the body's cells where it is either burned immediately as we run, walk or even think, or stored in the muscles and fat stores for later use. This happens with just about every food that contains carbohydrates, whether it is a plate of spinach or a plate of doughnuts. What differs is exactly how fast this reaction happens —and in very simple terms the glycemic index is a measure of that speed. Foods with a high glycemic index (known as high-GI foods) are converted rapidly to glucose, while foods with a low glycemic index (low-GI foods) are converted more slowly.

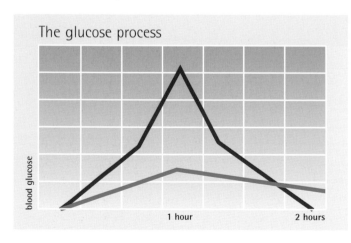

The glucose process

blood glucose

1 hour   2 hours

■ **High-GI foods** (such as white bread, baked potatoes, rice cakes, and watermelon) are converted into glucose quickly

■ **Low-GI foods** (such as peanuts, sausages, whole wheat spaghetti, and chocolate) are converted into glucose much more slowly

"Slowly does it"

Low-GI foods take longer to digest, so you feel full for longer

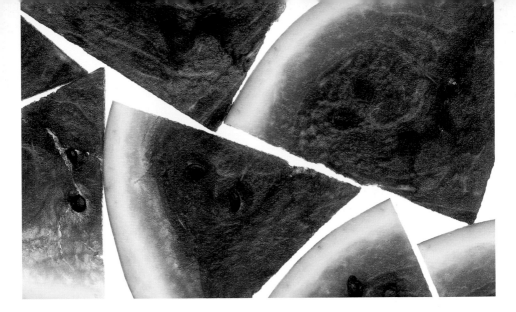

What has this got to do with our health?

The missing link is a hormone called insulin. When glucose is released into the bloodstream, it is the job of insulin to take it where it is needed. If the glucose is released slowly there is no problem—moderate levels of insulin are released and have time to "think" about where that glucose is needed most and send it there.

However, if high levels of glucose enter the bloodstream, the body panics. It might need glucose for fuel, but too much can be harmful. It therefore releases high levels of insulin which quickly transfer the glucose to the fat stores where it can do no harm. This can lead to weight gain if it happens too often.

But weight gain isn't the only consequence. If insulin levels are raised too often, the cells that normally respond to glucose become resistant to its signals. Less glucose is taken to where it is needed, and it remains in the bloodstream which causes cell damage, contributing to aging, and other problems such as furring of the arteries. And because the cells aren't getting enough fuel (which in itself causes fatigue), the body then triggers the release of more and more insulin to try to solve the problem. This boosts resistance further, and after many years can even trigger Type II diabetes.

Turning things around

Switching to a low-GI diet reverses this process. By ensuring you eat only foods that cause a gentle rise in glucose in your bloodstream, you prevent the panic reaction and balance your system. For healthy people this reduces the risk of insulin resistance occurring, and for the estimated 25 percent of people already suffering from the condition, it can give the cells enough of a break to allow them to resensitize. As you will see, the results can positively affect everything from your heart to your skin.

20 reasons
to eat low-GI foods

1 Researchers at Harvard University have shown that women who eat lots of refined carbohydrates have 10 percent less good cholesterol in their bloodstream, which keeps the heart healthy, and 76 percent more triglycerides (toxic fat), than low GI-dieters.

2 In a study at Yonsei University, in Seoul, South Korea, a group of men swapped white rice (high GI) for whole grains (low GI) and their levels of homocysteine (amino acid), fell by 28 percent in six weeks. High levels of homocysteine are linked to heart problems and can lead to Alzheimer's disease in later life.

3 A high fiber content is a contributing factor in making a food low GI. By increasing your intake of low-GI foods, you are more likely to get the 1 oz of daily recommended fiber. This may boost weight loss (fiber helps remove fat calories from the system), and may lower the risk of colon and other digestive cancers.

4 By not eating sugary foods you can look younger. Many dermatologists believe that refined carbohydrates cause skin inflammation. This creates high levels of free radicals (see page 39) which attack collagen and elastin fibers, causing wrinkles.

5 Reducing insulin levels helps acne and oily skin. Research from Colorado State University shows that high insulin levels lead to the release of higher levels of androgens (male hormones) triggering sebum production.

6 According to the World Health Organization, the number of people suffering from diabetes will double by 2030. Switching our high-GI diets to low-GI plans may cut numbers of potential sufferers greatly.

7 If you suffer from diabetes, a low-GI diet can help you control your condition more effectively. Eight out of the nine studies which have looked at the effects in diabetics of switching to a low-GI diet, have found that it helps keep blood glucose levels more stable.

8 A controversial theory by researchers at the University of Sydney suggests that high-GI diets are linked to short sight. The incidence of short sight is lower in the Pacific islands where high-GI foods are less common.

9 Sugary foods attack your immune system. When fighting illness, the average white blood cell destroys about 14 germs an hour. But, when exposed to 3½ oz of sugar that number falls to 1.4 germs per hour, and stays like that for two hours. Low-GI eating could cut the risks of cold and flu ailments.

10 A high-GI diet may increase the risk of breast cancer, as high insulin levels trigger an increase in insulin-like growth hormones, that encourage cancer cell growth.

11 An increased incidence of pancreatic cancer can be linked to a high-GI diet.

12 A low-GI diet can reduce the risk of stroke. Women who switched one serving of refined carbohydrates to whole grains each day cut their risk of stroke by 40 percent say researchers at Harvard.

13 Your energy levels rise dramatically when you go on a low-GI diet, as high-GI foods cause sudden peaks, then falls, in blood sugar causing energy levels to crash. The gentle rise that occurs with a low-GI diet creates a more steady energy flow.

14 You will have more stamina. Many exercisers think their bodies need high sugar bursts for fuel. In fact, eating a low-GI diet during training, gives better endurance.

15 Low-GI diets lead to happier people. A mental benefit of carbohydrates is that they boost levels of the calming hormone serotonin. High-GI carbohydrates create a quick mood boost, but a crash soon follows, leaving you grumpy and jittery. Low-GI foods prevent this rollercoaster effect.

16 Steady energy levels benefit your brain. In an average day, 40 percent of the glucose you make is used to power your brain. Low, steady doses of glucose from low-GI foods, improve attention span and memory.

17 Women can benefit from a low-GI diet as PMS (premenstrual syndrome) can be linked to erratic blood sugar levels. High-GI diets could be related to Polycystic Ovary Syndrome (PCOS) that can cause fertility problems. The ability of high insulin levels to increase levels of androgens (male hormones) in the body are believed to play a part here.

18 A low-GI diet may improve fertility. Imbalances in blood sugar can reduce the body's ability to handle the vital hormone, progesterone, for a successful pregnancy.

19 Children also benefit. Research has shown that children raised on diets high in refined sugars had lower IQs than those raised on low-GI diets. This could be due to the reduced level of nutrients in refined foods. High-GI eaters of any age have been shown to lack zinc, iron, folate, and calcium.

20 You may live longer. Studies show that people with high levels of vitamin C in their blood live up to 6 years longer than those with lower levels. A high-GI diet can decrease the amount of vitamin C you absorb by 25 percent. Glucose and vitamin C enter cells in the same way but if there is too much glucose, less vitamin C is absorbed.

What's your GI factor?

If you want to know whether you are at risk from health problems due to a high-GI diet, answer the following questions and find out.

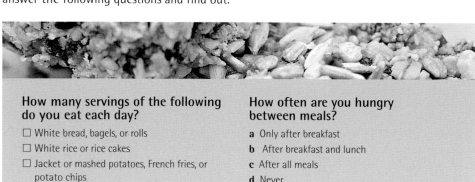

How many servings of the following do you eat each day?

☐ White bread, bagels, or rolls
☐ White rice or rice cakes
☐ Jacket or mashed potatoes, French fries, or potato chips
☐ Cakes
☐ Cookies
☐ Cornflakes, rice cereals, or honey-covered cereals

Score 1 point for every serving

When you eat vegetables, how likely are you to choose the following:

☐ Fava beans
☐ Parsnips
☐ Squash
☐ Rutabaga

Score 2 points for very likely, 1 point for occasionally, 0 points for never

Which of these is your most common breakfast?

a Cornflakes, rice cereals, or similar
b Toast and jelly
c Bacon and eggs
d Porridge and fruit

Score 2 points for a, 1 point for b, 0 points for c or d

How often are you hungry between meals?

a Only after breakfast
b After breakfast and lunch
c After all meals
d Never

Score 1 point for a, 2 points for b, 3 points for c, 0 points for d

If you gain weight, where does it tend to go on?

a Your stomach
b Your hips and thighs
c All over

Score 1 point for a, 0 points for b or c

How often do you get cravings for sugary snacks?

a Every day. I can set my watch by the 3pm chocolate run
b Only if I'm stressed, tired, or (for women) when I'm suffering PMS
c I never get cravings

Score 2 points for a, 1 point for b, 0 points for c

The results

More than 10 points

You are definitely on a high-GI diet and you may already be suffering some symptoms. Being hungry within an hour or so after eating is a sign of erratic blood sugar. Having sugar cravings around 3pm when our energy levels naturally dip, is another symptom. Gaining weight around your middle means that your fat stores are being controlled by insulin. Switch to a low-GI plan and see the benefits.

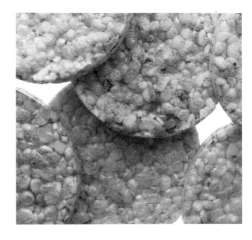

5–9 points

While you are on a lower-GI diet than those scoring higher points, there are still places where you could improve your diet to harness all the health benefits a low-GI diet may bring. Whether it is by switching to lower-GI versions of your favourite carbohydrate foods, or combining those healthy choices that you do make with ingredients that lower their GI, you can maximize weight loss efforts and help balance your mood, energy, and cravings for sweet foods.

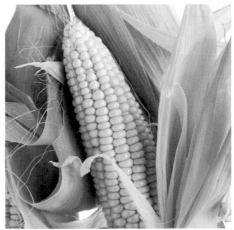

Less than 4 points

Well done; you are already likely to be eating a low-GI diet. However, you may not think you are harnessing all the benefits that this filling and healthy way of eating can bring. Perhaps you are not timing meals correctly, which is sapping your energy; or perhaps you are getting your portion sizes wrong, reducing the effects of your healthy choices. Whatever the reason, you can turn things around by following the advice that follows.

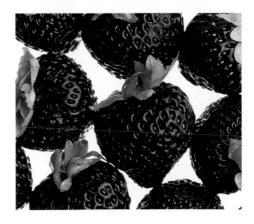

All foods are not equal

The whole premise of the GI diet is that some foods create a faster rise in insulin production than others. Therefore, by choosing low-GI foods instead of high-GI foods you can balance insulin levels and prevent weight gain.

Obviously, to do this you need to know which foods are the best to choose. A few years ago this was thought to be easy—it was believed that so-called complex carbohydrates (such as bread, pasta, and rice) were converted more slowly to glucose than simple carbohydrates (commonly thought of as the sweet sugars found in fruit, cakes, and cookies). However, the more we learn about the glycemic index, the more we realize that this isn't quite true. In fact, there are six main elements that determine the GI of a food:

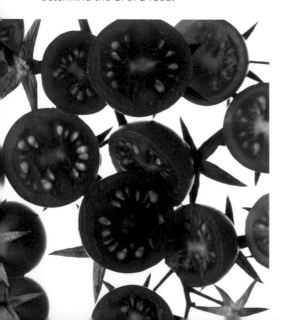

1 Does it contain carbohydrate?

Pure protein foods such as meat, fish, poultry, and eggs, and pure fats such as oils, butter, and margarine, contain no carbohydrate. As a result, the effect they have on glucose production is negligible. These foods are therefore low GI.

2 How much starch does it contain?

The easiest ingredient for our body to convert into glucose is starch. When foods are raw, this starch is generally found in hard, compact particles that the body finds hard to break down. However, if something disturbs these starch particles (for example, milling into flour), the body finds it much easier to digest them and they turn into glucose faster.

3 How much fiber does it contain?

Fiber slows the time it takes the body to break down a food. This is one reason why beans and legumes (which are wrapped in a fibrous shell) have such a low GI.

4 What kind of sugar does it contain?

There are four main types of sugar, and they raise blood sugar levels at different rates. Foods with a high concentration of glucose (such as sports drinks) need no conversion, so they raise blood sugar rapidly. Fructose (the sugar in fruit), however, converts slowly; as does lactose which is the main sugar in dairy products. This gives the majority of foods containing either fructose or lactose a low GI. The fourth sugar, sucrose, has a medium GI.

5 Does it contain fat?

As well as having no effect on glucose itself, fat slows the speed at which food leaves the stomach and reaches the liver, slowing glucose production. This is the reason why potato chips have a lower GI than most other types of potato.

6 How acidic is it?

Foods can contain acid ingredients—citrus fruits like oranges or lemons are a good example of this. The tang they create on your tongue comes from the citric acid they contain. Other acidic ingredients include lactic acid in milk products, and added ingredients, such as vinegars, in pickled products. Just like fat, acidity slows a food's progress through the system, and therefore slows the rate at which it converts into glucose.

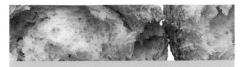

Some surprises

The combination of all the factors which affect a food's glycemic index can throw up some surprising results. In the GI world...

- **Parsnips** and **pineapple** can be fat-making foods
- **Peanuts** are better than **potatoes**
- **Bacon** is a diet food—**bagels** not so much
- **Chocolate** is equal to **cherries**
- **Watermelon** is as bad as **waffles**
- **French bread** should be eaten with as much care as **French fries**

But this doesn't mean you are restricted to a diet of nuts, bacon, and chocolate (as tasty as that might seem)—there is a whole host of GI-friendly foods for you to eat.

"Make the right choices"

By choosing low-GI foods, you can balance insulin levels and prevent weight gain

GI facts about carbohydrates

When you are following a low-GI diet, the biggest changes that are likely to occur are in the following six foods: bread, breakfast cereals, grains, pasta, potatoes, and rice. That is not just because they make up the majority of our diet, it is these foods that our body finds easiest to convert into glucose. But don't panic if you can't give up your bread and pasta—unlike high-protein diets, a low-GI diet doesn't ban starchy carbohydrates altogether from your eating plan. Instead, the idea is to switch your choices to those with the lowest impact on your blood sugar levels.

Bread

The average person eats around 2650 loaves of bread in their lifetime. Some days, it seems every meal we eat can contain some kind of bread product. This wouldn't be a problem if all of those were low-GI breads, but the majority aren't. They are often white breads, including baguettes, ciabatta and panini, made from extremely finely milled flour particles that take no time at all to break down into glucose. Switching from white breads to other choices is therefore a key GI-lowering tactic—and the easiest way to choose your new bread is to think of the three F's:

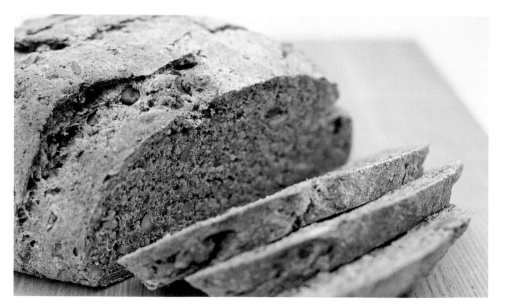

Fiber

The more fiber a bread contains, the lower its GI. If you really want to eat white or brown bread, choose one with added fiber. A much better choice, however, is multigrain or wholegrain breads which contain whole wheat grains. These not only boost the fiber content of the bread, but the hard husk around the wheat grains dramatically slows glucose conversion, making a low-GI food.

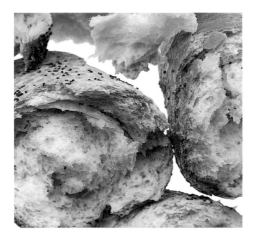

Finely ground—or not?

Most bread is produced by grinding the flour through steel grinders to produce very fine particles. Stoneground breads, however, are produced by crushing the wheat grains between two large stones to create larger, and less easily converted, particles—and therefore a lower GI.

Flour type

Choosing a bread made from an ingredient that has a lower GI than wheat leads to a more GI-friendly bread (see right).

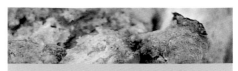

The good bread guide

Here is a guide to how quickly different bread types can raise glucose levels. At the top of the list are those that convert slowest—and are therefore good choices. Lower down are the rapid converters that should be avoided.

LOW GI
- **Barley bread** (with whole grains)
- **Soy bread**
- **Multigrain bread**
- **Rye and pumpernickel bread** (with whole grains)
- **Fruit bread**
- **Wheat tortillas**
- **White tortillas**
- **Sourdough bread**
- **Pita bread** (both white and brown)
- **Barley, rye, or pumpernickel bread** (without whole grains)
- **Stoneground white or brown bread**
- **White or brown bread** with added fiber
- **Brown or whole wheat bread or rolls**
- **White bread or rolls**
- **Bagels**
- **Gluten-free bread**

HIGH GI
- **Baguette**

Breakfast cereals

Breakfast is one of the most important meals of the day and shouldn't be skipped: studies show that regular breakfast eaters consume more nutrients and weigh less than those who don't eat it. This is partly because eating breakfast prevents the hunger pangs which could make you reach for a less nutritious mid-morning snack. However, this will only work if you eat the right kind of breakfast.

A high-GI breakfast cereal is just as likely to leave you hungry as no breakfast at all. When researchers at Tufts University in the USA fed volunteers a high-GI breakfast, they ate almost twice as many snack calories later in the day as those fed a low-GI one. Many breakfast cereals are high-GI as the high levels of processing alter the starch bonds, making them easy to break down. Also, many breakfast cereals have high levels of added sugar or honey, which raise their GI value.

High-fiber cereals are the best option as they are usually have a low GI rating and also have added health benefits.

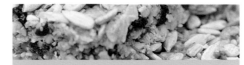

The good **breakfast** guide

LOW GI

Best choices
Noodle-shaped bran cereals (turning bran into a flake raises its GI), traditional porridge oats (not instant)

Moderate choices
Muesli

Best avoided
Honey cereals, sugary cereals, flaked cereals (bran, corn, or wheat), puffed cereals (wheat, corn, or rice), wheat biscuits, instant porridge.

HIGH GI

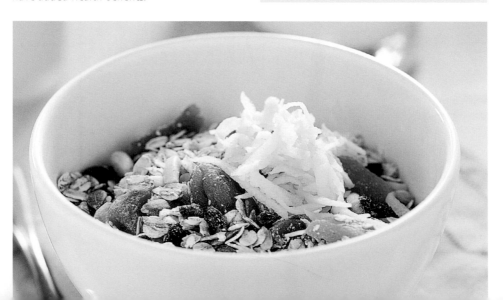

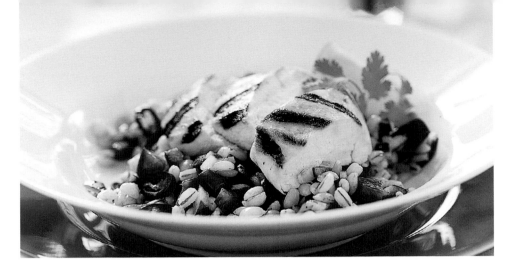

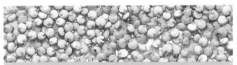

How to use grains

Most grains are simple to cook—just pop them into boiling water. The time they take to cook varies: barley can take 45 minutes, buckwheat takes 10–15 minutes, while couscous can be ready in as little as 3–4 minutes. Once cooked, they can be used in the following dishes:

- Use instead of potatoes or rice as a side dish alongside meat or vegetable dishes

- Add to stews, soups, or casseroles instead of potatoes or pasta to make a main meal

- Use as a great base for salads, helping to boost the fiber count and keep you feeling full for longer

- Use in flour form to make bread (look out for barley, buckwheat, and bulgar flours)

- Use in flake form as a breakfast cereal

Grains

It has been shown that when people start a low-GI diet, the variety of their diet increases by an average of nine new foods. The increased use of grains is one element of this, as many people tend to experiment more with grains rather than higher-GI staples such as rice and potatoes. It makes good health sense —most grains are high in essential B vitamins, and essential minerals like magnesium or phosphorus. Also, because they are subject to minimal processing, most grains have a low GI rating.

As grains are unfamiliar to many of us, here is a quick guide to what's what:

Barley (low GI)

Barley can be made into flour to create a very low-GI bread, and into flakes to make porridge. However, the best choice for a low-GI diet is the smooth ivory grains of pearl barley. Pearl barley is rather like a cross between white and brown rice in both flavor and texture.

Buckwheat (low GI)

This grain has a very nutty flavor and a strong taste which means it goes very well with meat or richly flavored vegetable dishes. You will sometimes see it called kasha, which is a roasted form of the whole grain.

Bulgar wheat (low GI)

If you have ever eaten the Middle Eastern salad tabbouleh, you have eaten bulgar wheat as it is the primary ingredient. Unlike other grains, bulgar wheat does not need cooking. It needs to be steeped in boiling water for about 30 minutes, or according to the instructions found on the package.

Couscous (medium GI)

This is made from semolina flour that has water added and is then rolled into tiny balls.

It is normally found in quick-cook varieties which need only minimal cooking or just soaking in water. This additional processing increases the GI count, but in small portions it is still a valid, healthy food for us to eat. It has a very mild flavor and is best accompanied by richly spiced or strongly flavored foods to enhance its flavor.

Millet (high GI)

The very small grains and relatively low protein count make millet a high-GI food. Use barley or bulgar wheat instead.

Quinoa (low GI)

Pronounced keen-wa, this nutty tasting grain from Peru is actually a fruit. It takes about 15 minutes to cook and the grains change from white to transparent when it is ready to eat.

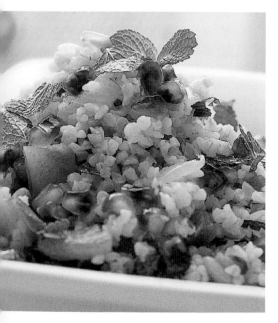 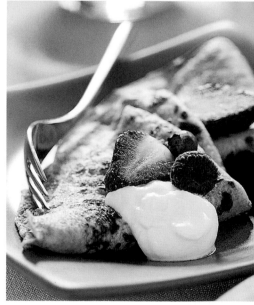

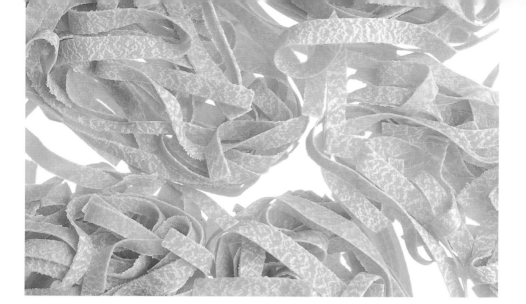

Pasta

Pasta is probably the food that confuses people most in the GI plan. On the face of it, it should be a high-GI food—it is packed with energy-giving carbohydrates, and in most cases it is a refined white food. However, virtually all pastas are low-GI foods because the flour used to make pasta (durum wheat) actually contains protein which slows its digestion in our bodies. Also, the starch particles in pasta are left fairly intact, which also slows things down.

One point to bear in mind with pasta, however, is that many of us eat much larger portions than is recommended—and the greater amount of any food you eat, the more glucose it will produce. To estimate a portion more easily, a standard 3 oz serving of spaghetti makes a bundle 1 inch across, while a similar serving of pasta shapes will fill half a cup. Also, the softer you cook your pasta the higher its GI index becomes—so it is better to stick to eating all your pasta dishes al dente. This means the pasta is slightly firm as you bite it.

Gluten-free pasta

The exception to the low-GI rule is gluten-free pasta. Made of wheat-free flour, gluten-free pasta doesn't have the protein protection that durum wheat provides.

Noodles

Some Asian noodles—udon, for example—are made from a more glutinous form of wheat flour than other types and this raises their GI rating. Rice noodles follow rice in having a high GI. Soba noodles, which are made from part buckwheat, part wheat, are a lower-GI choice. If you do want to eat noodles, choose glass noodles, also known as bean thread noodles, cellophane noodles and harusame noodles. These are made of beans and have a very low GI count.

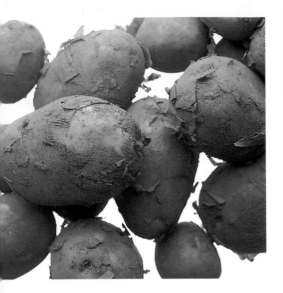

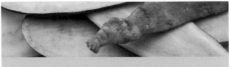

Yams or sweet potatoes?

These root vegetables are known by different names in different countries. Yams and sweet potatoes both have a low GI rating, so they are worth looking out for and including in your diet. Here's a brief guide to the differences between them:

• **Yams** are large vegetables with a thick, brown, knobbly skin, and a dry, white, purple or red flesh. They are usually found only in ethnic markets.

• **Sweet potatoes** are smaller, orange- or yellow-fleshed vegetables, with a thin orange or brown skin. They are sometimes known as kumura.

Potatoes

Despite being an excellent source of vitamin C, potassium, and the anti-aging nutrient glutathione, potatoes do score particularly poorly on the GI plan, with most varieties coming out as high-GI foods. The reason is believed to be because of their high starch content. However, new potatoes have a lower GI because they are picked earlier than other potatoes left on the plant to fully grow. This means that they have lower levels of starch when picked. New potatoes are therefore the only potatoes which have a low GI. Thus, it is much more beneficial to choose new potatoes for the majority of the meals you eat on the low-GI plan, or swap potatoes for some other form of low-GI carbohydrate.

There is an alternative option, try using sweet potatoes instead, which have a medium GI and can be roasted, mashed or chipped in just the same way as regular potatoes. Sweet potatoes actually provide even more nutrients than a normal potato. In fact, when the US Center for Science in the Public Interest ranked vegetables in order of their content of fiber and six vital nutrients (vitamins A and C, folate, iron, copper, and calcium) sweet potatoes came out top of the lot. This makes them a great food to eat.

Yams are also a good potato substitute and have a slightly lower GI, but they don't contain as many vitamins as sweet potatoes.

Rice

The GI content of rice depends primarily on which of two types of starch it contains—amylose, which is tightly bonded together, or amylopectin, which is more branched out. Because of its tight bonds, amylose tends not to break down as easily as amylopectin, so types of rice high in amylose have a lower GI than those high in amylopectin.

So how do you tell which your rice is? The theory is that if the grains stick together it is a high-GI rice; if they don't it is a lower one. However, the new easy-cook rices have made this test almost impossible for anyone but a rice expert to use. It is simpler to remember to choose those types of rice with a medium-GI content (see right).

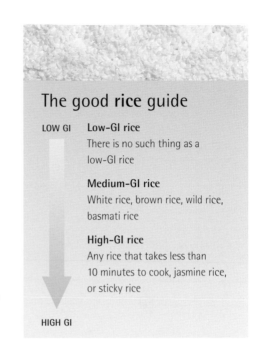

The good **rice** guide

LOW GI

Low-GI rice
There is no such thing as a low-GI rice

Medium-GI rice
White rice, brown rice, wild rice, basmati rice

High-GI rice
Any rice that takes less than 10 minutes to cook, jasmine rice, or sticky rice

HIGH GI

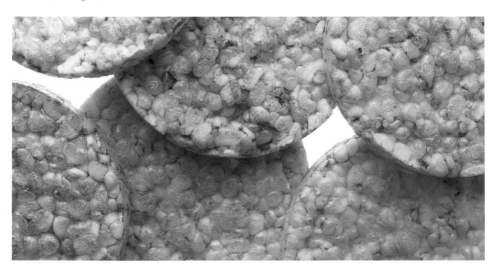

"Sticky or not?"

The theory is that if rice grains stick together, it is a high-GI rice, if they don't it is a low one

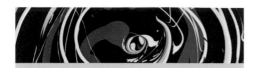

Chocolate—a paradox

Chocolate has a low GI because of its high concentration of dairy products, its high fat content, and the fact that it contains sucrose which is relatively slow to be converted into glucose. On top of this, chocolate is actually quite a healthy food as it contains high levels of antioxidants, as many as heart-healthy red wine. As a result, a little chocolate is allowed on the low-GI diet.

Remember, though, that added sugar-based ingredients like caramel or nougat will cause the GI to rise from low to medium. It's always best to stick to simple chocolate bars—particularly those made from dark chocolate.

Carbohydrate snacks

We have become a snacking generation—in Europe alone, 1.4 million tonnes of snacks are eaten each year, while in the USA almost one-fifth of daily calories come from snack foods such as cookies, cakes, chocolate, and potato chips. This is bad news as most snacks have a high GI—and the constant drip, drip, drip of sugar into the system is a major cause of increased insulin levels.

When it comes down to it, most sugary snacks (cakes, waffles, doughnuts, scones) have a high GI. Others, like cookies or muffins, have a medium GI. But all contain high levels

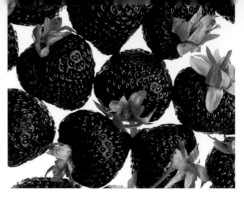

of harmful fats called transfats (see page 35). It would be sad to include these foods in a diet with as many heart-friendly health benefits as eating low GI.

Savory snacks

A snack doesn't need to be sweet to raise glucose levels too quickly. Rice cakes, for example, a staple snack for the health conscious, have a very high GI because the rice is processed to make it into biscuit form and the starch particles become extremely easy to break down. Pretzels and popcorn suffer the same fate. Potato chips have only a medium GI because their high fat content slows their conversion. However, they too suffer from the bad-fat problem (see page 35).

What you can eat

This doesn't mean snacking is banned completely when you are eating a low-GI diet. In fact, it is encouraged—eating a small meal or snack every two hours keeps blood sugar levels even more stable than eating three large meals a day. You just need to choose the right foods. Those that do fit the low-GI, healthy fat principle include nuts, seeds, fruit, yogurt, and chocolate.

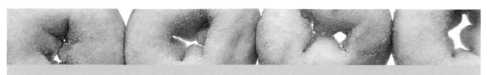

Carbohydrates at a glance

Low-GI carbohydrates

Breads Multigrain bread and rolls, barley breads, rye or pumpernickel bread with grains, soy bread, wheat tortilla wraps

Cereals Bran strands, porridge

Grains Barley, bulgar wheat, buckwheat, quinoa

Pasta and noodles Egg noodles or glass noodles (cellophane or bean thread noodles)

Potatoes New potatoes, yams

Rice There are no low-GI rices

Sweet snacks Milk, dark or white chocolate, yogurt, low-fat ice cream

Savory snacks Nuts and seeds

Medium-GI carbohydrates

Breads Barley, rye or pumpernickel bread (no grains), brown bread, fruit bread, pita bread, sourdough bread, white tortilla wraps, white or brown bread with added fiber, stoneground bread

Cereals Bran cereal with fruit, muesli (low sugar and regular varieties), wheat cereal

Grains Couscous

Pasta and noodles All types of pasta, soba noodles, udon noodles

Potatoes Chips, sweet potatoes

Rice Basmati, brown, risotto, white, wild

Sweet snacks Cookies, chocolate bars containing caramel or nougat, ice cream

Savory snacks Potato chips, corn chips

High-GI carbohydrates

Breads Bagels, baguettes, gluten-free bread, white bread and rolls

Cereals Flaked cereals (corn, wheat, or bran), honey-coated cereals, puffed cereals, instant porridge

Grains Millet

Pasta and noodles Gluten-free pasta, rice noodles

Potatoes Baked, French fries, mashed (real or instant)

Rice Fast-cook varieties, jasmine rice, sticky rice

Sweet snacks Hard candy, doughnuts, jelly beans, chewy fruit candy, waffles

Savory snacks Popcorn, pretzels, rice cakes

GI facts about
fruit and vegetables

These vital health foods are a major part of any low-GI diet—and here's why.

Fruit

As a general rule, fruit is a low-GI food. This might surprise you as it usually tastes sweet, and it is digested very quickly. However, the fact that the main sugar in many fruits is fructose gives us a major metabolic advantage, as it has to be converted into glucose before it can be used by your body. This prevents the sudden peak in blood sugar that can cause rapid insulin release.

What affects the GI of a fruit?

Acidity Generally, the more acidic a fruit is, the lower its glycemic index. This is good news for fans of sour fruit like grapefruit, lemons, and limes. However, many sweet fruits, such as kiwi fruit and oranges, also have high acidity.

Fiber content Fruits are also high in soluble fiber, the type that has been shown to lower GI count. Generally, fruits with the highest soluble fiber content (apples and pears, for example, that are high in the fiber pectin) are those with the lowest GI. Pectin is also known to be an appetite-suppressor.

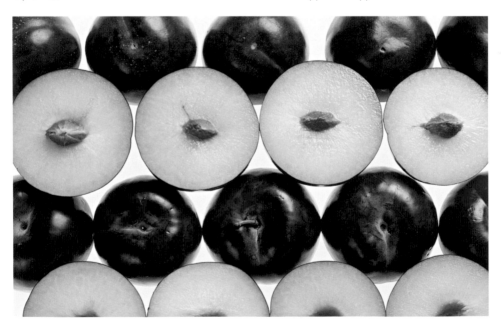

Fructose content Fruits generally contain a mixture of three sugars: fructose, sucrose, and glucose. The more fructose (and less glucose) a fruit contains, the lower its GI count. This is why watermelon, which is high in glucose, has a higher GI than other fruits.

Processing The processing involved with canning fruit alters its make-up, softening the fibrous strands within it. This makes the fruit easier to break down and slightly increases the rate at which glucose is created. Many fruits are canned in syrup which can contain fast-release sugars, and raise GI from a low to medium rating. Fruit juice also has a higher GI than the fruit it was extracted from as the fiber has been removed. Dried fruit generally raises blood sugar faster than the raw fruit it is made from.

Vegetables

Like fruit, the majority of vegetables are low-GI foods. This is because, despite the fact that many are classed as carbohydrate foods, the actual amount of carbohydrates they contain is very small—and in most cases, they are not types that cause rapid rises in blood sugar. On top of this, the fact that most vegetables are very high in fiber, a known GI-inhibitor, means that most vegetables can be seen as a free food on a low-GI diet.

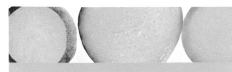

The good fruit guide

LOW GI

Low-GI fruits
Apples, dried apricots, avocado, blackberries, blueberries, cherries, grapefruit, white grapes, kiwi fruit, citrus fruits, peaches (fresh and canned in juice), pears (fresh and canned in juice), plums, prunes, raspberries, strawberries, tomatoes

Medium-GI fruits
Apricots (fresh and canned), bananas, cantaloupe melon, figs (fresh and dried), red grapes, mango, papaya, peaches (canned in syrup), pears (canned in syrup), raisins

High-GI fruits
Watermelon, dates

HIGH GI

"Low-carb, high-fiber"

Most vegetables can be seen as a free food on a low-GI diet

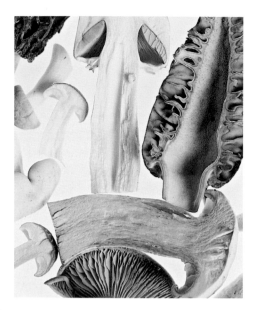

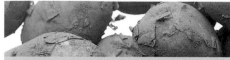

The good **vegetable** guide

LOW GI | **Low-GI vegetables**
Alfalfa, artichokes, arugula, asparagus, bean sprouts, broccoli, Brussels sprouts, carrots, cabbage, cauliflower, celery, cucumber, eggplant, endive, fennel, garlic, green beans, kale, leeks, lettuce, mushrooms, okra, onions, peas, radicchio, radish, snow pea, spinach, sweet peppers, Swiss chard, watercress, zucchini

Medium-GI vegetables
Beet, corn, corn kernels

High-GI vegetables
Parsnips, rutabaga, squash,
HIGH GI | turnips

There are, however, some exceptions to this—notably starchy root vegetables such as beet, parsnips, and rutabaga, or sweet vegetables like squash, which are medium- or high-GI foods. In fact, parsnips have a higher GI than jelly beans.

This doesn't mean that beet and parsnips are banned forever, though. One of the criticisms of the glycemic index is the way that it is measured. To determine a food's GI, researchers measure a serving of the food that contains 50 g of carbohydrate. And it takes a very large quantity of parsnip or beet to give you 50 g of carbohydrate. If you eat less than this, and you will, the reaction will not be as severe. So, as long as portions are kept moderate, and you don't eat them for every meal, there is no reason to completely ban high-GI vegetables from your diet entirely.

Cooking and processing vegetables

In all cases, the glycemic index is slightly raised when vegetables are cooked or processed—but the change is so minimal it won't make a huge difference to your blood sugar levels. After all, some vegetables are more nutritious when cooked, canned, or frozen. For example, we get three times more betacarotene from cooked carrots than raw ones as heat softens the tough cell walls, making it easier for us to absorb the goodness within. Pumpkin, green beans, and broccoli are also more nutritious when frozen or canned.

GI facts about protein foods

The principal factor in determining the glycemic index of a food is whether or not it contains carbohydrates. Pure protein foods, such as meat, fish, and poultry, contain no carbohydrate and so have a low GI. However, there are some foods that contain high levels of protein, but also some level of carbohydrate, and therefore have a higher GI rating.

Beans and legumes

Most of us don't eat enough of these vital health foods—but we should. A diet that contains regular servings of legumes has been shown to lead to lower cholesterol levels, to help balance hormones in women, possibly reducing the risk of breast cancer. And, according to researchers at Australia's Monash University, legumes are the number one protector of longevity.

In terms of the GI diet, beans and legumes are also great foods, as most of them have a low GI due to the fibrous coating around them which slows conversion. Don't forget also that these foods don't just have a low GI in their natural form—tofu and other meat-replacement products made from soybeans, hummus or falafel made from chickpeas, and soups or dhal made from lentils all have a low GI count as well.

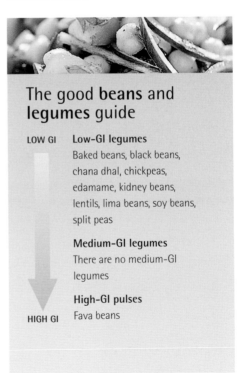

The good **beans** and legumes guide

LOW GI

Low-GI legumes
Baked beans, black beans, chana dhal, chickpeas, edamame, kidney beans, lentils, lima beans, soy beans, split peas

Medium-GI legumes
There are no medium-GI legumes

High-GI pulses
Fava beans

HIGH GI

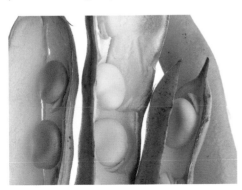

Watch points

As with all processed products, the amount of sugar added to a food will vary—and increase its GI count. Soy milk, for example, commonly has sugar added. **To ensure you are using a low-GI product, choose brands with less than 4 g of carbohydrate per 1 cup serving.** This will be listed on the product's nutrition label, and most good brands will be labeled "unsweetened."

Another area that can alter GI is the addition of coatings, such as bread crumbs or batter, to protein foods like chicken or fish, or the wheat used to bulk out burgers and sausages. Although amounts are usually so small that the difference is negligible, pure protein foods are healthier.

Dairy products

Again, while many of us believe these to be pure protein foods, the sugar lactose which many dairy products contain will be converted into glucose in the body. The good news is that these sugars are converted slowly, making dairy foods like milk, cheese, yogurt—and even low-fat ice cream—low-GI food choices. The only exception to this rule is condensed milk which commonly has other sugars added to it, but this is unlikely to be a staple part of your diet.

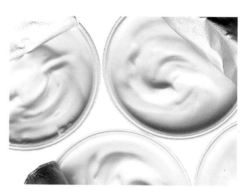

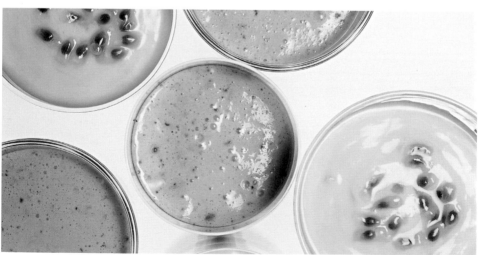

Nuts and seeds

The combination of protein and fats gives nuts and seeds their low GI—but this isn't the only reason these foods are recommended as part of the low-GI plan. They are also vital sources of the healthy fats our bodies need to stay healthy, look good—and even lose weight. To convince you of their health benefits even further, a study showed that people eating 5 oz of nuts each week were associated with living longer than those who did not eat them.

Some nutritionists describe seeds as a superfood, citing the fact that if a plant can grow from a seed, imagine what a powerhouse of nutrients and energy it must contain within. Nuts like peanuts, cashews, brazils, or walnuts, and seeds like pumpkin or sunflower can easily be eaten by the handful as a snack or be sprinkled over salads. Also remember that spreads and dips made from nuts or seeds, such as peanut butter and tahini, will also have a low GI and can make great alternatives to butter or margarine. If you are watching your weight, though, remember nuts and seeds can be calorific.

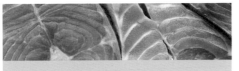

Pure proteins

All of the following foods can be seen as free foods on a low-GI diet (though watch fat counts carefully if you are dieting, or want to improve heart health).

Anchovies	Halibut	Shrimp
Angler fish	Ham	Skate
Bacon	Kippers	Sole
Beef	Lamb	Squid
Chicken	Liver	Swordfish
Clams	Lobster	Trout
Cod	Mackerel	Tuna
Crab	Mussels	Veal
Duck	Pilchards	Venison
Eggs	Pork	
Flounder	Salmon	
Goose	Sardines	
Haddock	Sea bass	

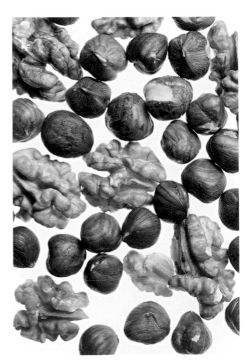

Drinks

It is not just solid food that turns to glucose in our systems—drinks do too. It is easy to consume them and forget about their potential effects on our health and weight. Choosing low-GI drinks is just as important as low-GI foods.

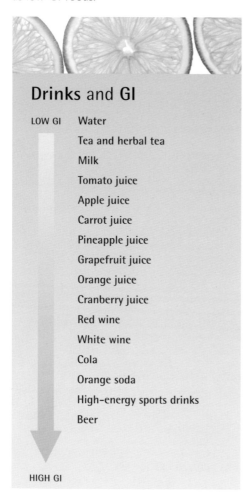

Drinks and GI

LOW GI

Water

Tea and herbal tea

Milk

Tomato juice

Apple juice

Carrot juice

Pineapple juice

Grapefruit juice

Orange juice

Cranberry juice

Red wine

White wine

Cola

Orange soda

High-energy sports drinks

Beer

HIGH GI

A note about coffee

Recent research from the Netherlands has revealed that the caffeine in coffee can actually increase the chance of cells becoming resistant to insulin—therefore increasing the amount your body is likely to secrete. As a result, caffeine is not a very good choice for a low-GI diet.

The problem is that many of us can actually become addicted to caffeine—and when we stop our intake we can suffer headaches. However, if you wean off caffeine slowly you can quit altogether without suffering any symptoms. To do this, replace one-quarter of each cup of coffee you have each day with decaffeinated. Do this for three days, which is how long it takes your body to become accustomed to the new level. On the fourth day, replace another quarter of the cup with decaffeinated. Repeat until you are drinking no caffeine at all, which should take around 12 days.

Alcoholic drinks

Alcoholic spirits, such as gin, vodka, and whiskey, are also best avoided. Although they have very little effect on insulin—and are therefore technically low GI—a high intake of spirits is linked to other health problems.

Red wine is a better choice than spirits. Although it has a medium GI value, it contains antioxidants, which are good for your heart.

The fat factor

Many high-fat foods—chocolate, nuts, meat, dairy products, for example—are also low-GI. This is because fat does not raise blood sugar levels. In order to be healthy, a low-GI diet needs to include the right types of fat.

Why some fat is good for you

Fat is essential for a healthy body. For starters, without it you wouldn't be able to process the fat-soluble vitamins A, D, E, and K which help keep your eyes, bones, skin, and brain healthy and fully functioning. Your body uses fat for energy, and to create healthy cells and hormones, which regulate everything from how we feel pain to women's menstrual cycles. Without some fat your body won't look or feel good, but you need to make sure you are getting the right types.

Types of fat

Foods can contain four types of fat: saturated, monounsaturated, polyunsaturated, and hydrogenated. (Also known as transfats, hydrogenated fats are made when vegetable oils are processed into a solid fat through heating.) When you eat a food that contains fat, you take in the first three of above fats, and occasionally the fourth. What varies is the percentage of different fats the food contains: meat for example is higher in saturated fat than it is in polyunsaturated fat; oily fish is

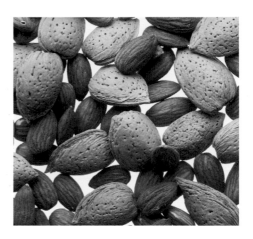

just the opposite. It is this ratio, plus the presence of transfats, that determines whether we think a food is "healthy" or not. On a low-GI diet, you're aiming to choose not only low-GI foods for the majority of your meals—but when those foods also contain fats, to pick those high in healthy fats rather than unhealthy ones.

The foods to choose

Focusing on foods containing healthy fats and minimizing intakes of unhealthy ones is the key to good health. The GI plan makes this simple as many of the foods that contain saturated fat are also high in sugar so are already a banned food. However, you should always remove any obvious fat from low-GI foods such as red meat, avoid frying your food, and choose low-fat dairy options wherever possible.

When low GI meets high

While it won't do any harm to eat only low-GI foods, after a while life could get a bit monotonous. This brings us to the best news of all about a low-GI Diet—no food is completely banned. But if you eat a high-GI food, follow the rules below to reduce its effect on your blood sugar.

The rules

1 **When you eat a high-GI food, watch your portion size.** Scientists calculate the glycemic index of food by feeding a volunteer the amount of the food that contains 50 g of carbohydrate. For celery, this amount is about 50 sticks, for cooked rice it is 5 oz, and for sugar it is 4 tablespoons. The more you eat, the greater the amount of glucose will be produced; by eating less, you'll create less. Control your high-GI portion sizes and you'll control the amount of sugar produced.

2 **Every time you eat a high-GI food, eat at least two low-GI foods of the same, or a larger, quantity.** This lowers the average GI of a meal and decreases the glucose produced. In an ideal world, one of those foods would be a protein food like meat, poultry, fish, eggs, legumes, nuts, or dairy. The other would be fruit or vegetables. Therefore, if you have ½ cup high-GI cornflakes for breakfast,

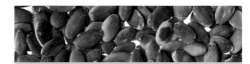

Low-GI **portions** for high-GI foods

Potatoes 4 oz

Rice ½ cup cooked weight (roughly 2 tablespoons dried)

Bread 1–2 slices

Breakfast cereals ½ cup

Root vegetables 4 oz

Popcorn and pretzels ½ cup

accompany this with ½ cup of skimmed milk and a sliced peach.

3 **Don't eat more than one high-GI food or two medium-GI foods a day.** Ideally have less. While these rules make eating high-GI foods less damaging to your system, to allow your body to get back into balance, skip high-GI foods as often as possible.

4 **If the meal allows, add something acidic.** Food with integrated acid slows its conversion to glucose, so does acid added to high-GI food. The acid factor can reduce the GI of some high-sugar foods by 30 percent.

The GI pyramid

There is a huge range of foods that you can eat on a low-GI plan, but how much of each food should you eat each day? The traditional food pyramid, which most of us regard as being healthy, focuses primarily on starchy carbohydrates like bread, pasta, and rice, recommending up to 11 servings a day. Even if you stuck to the lowest-GI versions of these foods, there would still be a lot of glucose within your system. Follow the GI-friendly pyramid to help you with your eating plan.

Tailor-made diets

If you are not going to follow our specific diet plan, use the pyramid as a guide to giving back your body the balance it craves. And don't forget to follow these essential guidelines:

• **Remember all carbohydrates are not equal.** If you do nothing else, at least switch high-GI carbohydrate foods like white rice, white bread, sugary cereals, and potatoes for lower-GI choices.

• **Eat at least three meals a day.** Skipping meals can often lead to a drop in blood sugar that trigger cravings for high-GI foods. It is a good idea to include two low-GI snacks each day as well.

• **If you do eat a high-GI food, follow the guidelines opposite** to reduce its effects on your body.

• **Remember fat is still bad for your body.** Choose foods that are low in saturated fat for most meals and include foods containing heart-healthy fats.

• **Drinks count.** Don't undo all your low-GI eating by washing it down with sugary sodas, fruit drinks, or alcohol. If you do drink alcohol, stick to safe drinking limits.

The pyramid guide

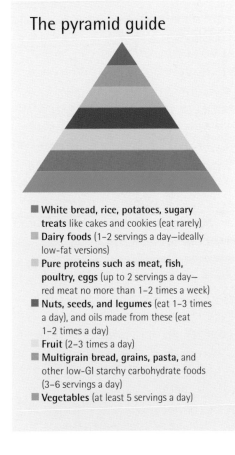

■ **White bread, rice, potatoes, sugary treats** like cakes and cookies (eat rarely)
■ **Dairy foods** (1–2 servings a day—ideally low-fat versions)
■ **Pure proteins such as meat, fish, poultry, eggs** (up to 2 servings a day—red meat no more than 1–2 times a week)
■ **Nuts, seeds, and legumes** (eat 1–3 times a day), and oils made from these (eat 1–2 times a day)
■ **Fruit** (2–3 times a day)
■ **Multigrain bread, grains, pasta,** and other low-GI starchy carbohydrate foods (3–6 servings a day)
■ **Vegetables** (at least 5 servings a day)

GI ways to boost health

Many studies have shown that what we eat affects our health. Fruit, vegetables, whole grains, and legumes emerge as vital health protectors. Follow any low-GI diet (which will be high in all of these), and you can harness the protective power of food, lose weight, and boost energy.

GI for weight loss

The point of the low-GI plan is to stop the rapid release of glucose into the system and decrease insulin production. This affects your weight. Insulin stops excess sugar being pushed into fat stores and lessens appetite, as insulin is an appetite stimulant. When insulin levels fall, the body releases glucagon into the system.

Glucagon's job is to remove glucose from fat stores and burn it as fuel. The more often glucagon is released into your system, the more fat you burn. Eating low-GI foods keeps insulin levels low, and by cutting calories you maximize the chances of glucagon being produced and putting your body into fat-burning mode. This makes for more successful weight loss—but when you eat low-GI you get other slimming benefits too.

Fill-up factor

You are less likely to be hungry on a low-GI diet than a high-GI one. When US researchers fed volunteers a low-GI meal, they ate 81 percent less calories at their next meal than those fed a high-GI meal. This is because the appetite-increasing effects of insulin are suppressed in low-GI foods, and also low-GI meals tend to be higher in fiber and protein, making you feel fuller.

Craving control

Sugar cravings can derail the most determined dieter—but they are far less likely to occur on a low-GI plan as you don't experience sudden rises and falls in blood sugar levels.

Vital vitamins

Some studies have suggested that people who eat a high-GI diet are lacking zinc, calcium, iron, and vitamin C. All of these are vital fat-burning nutrients. Maximize weight loss by going low-GI, and increasing your intake of these fat fighters.

Burning boost

Low-GI diets tend to be high in fiber, which slows down digestion and moderates blood sugar levels. For every gram of fiber you eat, your body burns 7 kcal (29 kj) to process it as it travels through your digestive system. By eating 1 oz of the daily recommended fiber you can burn up to 200 kcal (840 kj).

GI for anti-aging

There's no doubt that eating a low-GI diet helps your health: reduced risk of diabetes, heart disease and some forms of cancer have been linked to a lowered intake of high-GI foods. The reasons why are to do with sugar.

Soft, white—and deadly

Sugar is a naturally sticky substance—and particles of glucose in the blood are no exception. If sugar is left in the bloodstream rather than being processed into fuel that can be burnt as energy, particles can stick to protein cells, a process called cross-linking.

The collagen fibers that run through our bodies are prone to cross-linking. Fibers lose flexibility, become brittle and break down. In the skin, this leads to wrinkles, in joints to a lack of mobility. In the lungs it leads to a decreased lung capacity and less oxygenation of the tissues, and in the blood vessels it leads to a stiffening, making the heart work harder. These effects are the main signs of aging.

Sugary foods also increase the number of free radicals in your system. When US researchers at Buffalo University gave volunteers a meal containing 300 kcal (1260 kj) of sugar, their free radicals increased by 140 percent—more than when they ate a meal full of fat.

Time to fight back

Free radicals are atoms containing electrons that are missing a "partner electron," and are the main cause of aging and illness. They steal electrons from other atoms in the body. As this

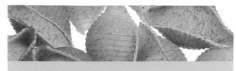

GI for energy

The rapid insulin rise that is triggered by high-GI foods means the glucose in our blood is rapidly pushed into the fat stores. Thus the glucose that should have gone to feed our muscles—and more importantly our brains—isn't used. This creates a lack of fuel, resulting in low energy. If you then reach for more sugary carbohydrates, the problem is compounded further.

Carbohydrates also contain substances that the brain converts to a chemical called serotonin. This helps calm the body and creates a sense of wellbeing—in small doses. If large doses of serotonin are produced by eating a lot of high-GI carbohydrates, we can feel very sleepy.

By eating a low-GI diet you can change this. Because the body isn't subjected to sudden surges in sugar, it doesn't experience sudden falls either, keeping energy more constant and reducing cravings for more carbohydrates. This means your serotonin levels are kept under control, allowing you to harness the stress-relieving benefits of serotonin without feeling the negative effects of overload.

happens, healthy cells get damaged, leading to aging or changes in the cell that trigger disease. By following a low-GI diet with less sugar, fewer free radicals are released into your system, slowing the ageing process.

Genius weight-loss plan

This easy-to-follow plan does the hard work for you. Each day has a calculated calorie count, so all you have to do is simply follow the menus.

One of the major benefits of low-GI eating is that it is a great way to lose weight. No food is banned, so you don't get as many diet-destroying cravings. Most importantly, however, you actually rebalance the system of your body that controls fat storage and fat burning, ensuring the calories you cut really do end up as weight lost. Whether you want to lose a little or a lot, your slim new shape starts here.

The low-GI plan

By following the low-GI plan you'll quickly discover how much better you can feel. It will help you lose a few pounds and boost your everyday energy levels.

The Genius weight-loss plan (see pages 40–71) will show you how to lose weight the GI way. Just follow the daily meal plans, already mapped out for you on the following pages. Feel energized by following the energy rules. By using the principles of low-GI eating you can also boost your immune system, too.

Using the weight-loss plan

Once you have the right mindset, losing weight is just a matter of burning more calories than you eat. The key to success is working out how many calories you need to eat in a day to create a safe calorie deficit. It is not a case of the more you cut a day, the better. By cutting too many calories your body will slow down your metabolism, reducing the amount of calories you burn. It is recommended that you cut only 500 kcal (2100 kj) from your daily intake. You will lose 1 lb each week—which may sound slow, but means you won't be hungry, you can eat treats like chocolate, you are more likely to lose fat than muscle—and the weight is more likely to stay off.

The diet plan on the pages that follow provide 1500 kcal (6300 kj) a day. This is the amount the average 154 lb woman in a sedentary job would need to lose weight. If you weigh more, or are more active, increase the amount of calories each day—if you weigh less, you'll need to decrease them. This is easy with the help of the GI charts (see pages 75–93). Don't swap meals from different days, as each day has a set calorie count.

Exercise

Exercise is relevant when eating a low-GI diet as it decreases the insulin sensitivity of the cells, speeding up the rate at which your body starts producing glucagon. Each week aim to do at least 2 hours of exercise. You can plan your own activities, but the program details an exercise task for each day.

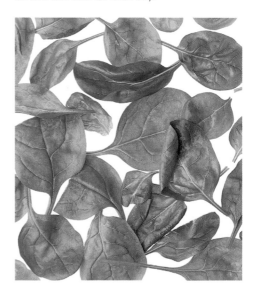

The eating for energy rules

Not only will you be focusing on low-GI foods, you will also be tailoring the timing of those foods to ensure that they give the most benefits to your body. This means following these four simple rules:

1 **Always eat a fiber-filled breakfast.** Any breakfast refills energy stores used up overnight, but a fiber-filled breakfast also helps boost the digestion, making it easier to absorb energy-giving nutrients from other foods. It will also prevent constipation, which is a major cause of fatigue.

2 **Add protein to every meal.** This creates even slower-burning energy, and helps counteract the negative effects of too many carbohydrates. Protein is particularly important at lunch. Our energy levels naturally dip around 3pm. If you eat a high-carbohydrate meal for lunch, this natural dip combines with sugar dips and serotonin boosts to create fatigue.

3 **Focus on carbohydrates in the evening.** By eating a more carbohydrate-heavy meal in the evening, you produce serotonin when you need it most—before bedtime. This helps ensure a more restful night's sleep and less fatigue the next day.

4 **Eat small meals every four hours.** Digestion takes its toll, and eating large meals can be tiring. Eating three small meals and two or three snacks a day prevents this.

Calculating your recommended intake

First calculate your basal metabolic rate (BMR). To do this, multiply your weight in pounds by 10. This is roughly how many calories (kcal) or kilojoules (kj) you burn a day while at rest.

Of course most of us don't spend all day lying on the sofa so, depending on how active you are, you need to multiply that figure further.

- **Sedentary job** (office work) **x 1.3**
- **Moderately active job** (shop worker, homemaker) **x 1.4**
- **Active job** (postperson, nurse) **x 1.5**
- **Very active job** (builder, fitness trainer, courier) **x 1.7**

This gives the total amount of energy you burn on an average day. You should be eating 500 kcal (2100 kj) less than this to lose 1 lb of weight a week.

You should eat at least three energy-giving foods a day, such as breakfast cereals, beans and legumes, oily fish, citrus fruit and berries, red meat and green leafy vegetables.

You will also see that, unlike other weight-loss plans, this diet doesn't have serving sizes. Eat enough so you feel full, but not overfull.

Day 1

This is your first day on the road to a slim new shape. The main thing you will notice is that you won't get hungry—in fact you may be eating more food than you would normally do. Don't panic and don't skip meals—eating regularly fires up your metabolism and actually increases the amount of weight you can lose.

Breakfast
Bowl of porridge
Use ¾ cup rolled oats and make according to package instructions. Top with a large handful of blueberries, strawberries, or sliced peaches instead of sugar
Glass of unsweetened orange juice
⅔ cup

Snack
Small carton of low-fat fruit yogurt ½ cup
Handful of dried apricots 2 oz

Lunch
Moroccan tomato and chickpea salad (see recipe, right)
Broiled chicken breast 5 oz
ALTERNATIVE:
Broiled chicken breast sandwich
5 oz chicken breast served on barley, multigrain or soy bread, topped with sliced tomato and a little mustard
large salad of celery, cucumber, and shredded carrot

Snack
1 banana
10 brazil nuts

Dinner
Broiled tuna steak
5 oz of tuna topped with 1 serving of Tomato and Sweet Pepper Salsa (see recipe, bottom right) or 2 tablespoons of prepared salsa. Serve with 4 oz of new potatoes and 3 oz of snow peas

Get a breath of fresh air

Take a 30-minute walk at your own pace. Aim for a level that gets you slightly out of breath, however, as this will burn more calories and strengthen your heart and lungs. To make it more fun, take a friend and walk round the local park catching up on the latest news.

Calories burnt: 150

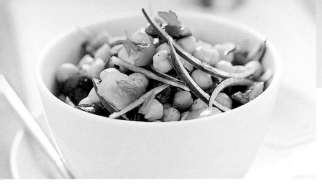

NUTRITION TIP

Chickpeas are a great source of fiber and rich in magnesium and folate. Eating them regularly can lower the risk of heart disease and diabetes.

Moroccan tomato and chickpea salad

Preparation time 10 minutes, plus standing   **Serves** 4

1 red onion, finely sliced

13 oz cans chickpeas, drained and rinsed

4 tomatoes, chopped

4 tablespoons lemon juice

1 tablespoon olive oil

handful of herbs (such as mint and parsley), chopped

pinch of paprika

pinch of ground cumin

salt and pepper

• Simply mix together all the ingredients in a large non-metallic bowl and set aside for 10 minutes to allow the flavors to infuse, then serve.

kcal 200 (840 kj)   **protein** 12 g   **carbohydrate** 30 g   **fat** 5 g   **GI** L

Tomato and sweet pepper salsa

Preparation time 10 minutes, plus standing   **Serves** 4

4 tomatoes, finely chopped

1 green chili, finely chopped

1 red bell pepper, cored, seeded, and finely chopped

grated zest and juice of 1 lime

2 tablespoons chopped parsley

• Mix together all the ingredients in a small bowl. Leave for 10 minutes to infuse, then serve.

kcal 12 (50 kj)   **protein** 0.6 g   **fat** negligible   **carbohydrate** 2.6 g   **GI** L

Day 2

The key to a diet's success is sticking with it. Before you begin today, look back at what went well and what didn't yesterday. Now look at why things went wrong, and what could stop them recurring. This analysis helps you to develop slimming safety nets that mean you won't fall into the same traps.

Breakfast

Glass of unsweetened orange juice ⅔ cup
2 slices of toast
Choose multigrain, barley or soy bread and spread with 2 teaspoons of ricotta cheese and 2 teaspoons of all-fruit conserve such as blackberry

Snack

Protein shake
made from 2 scoops of whey protein powder mixed with water, and 4 oz of tinned peaches in natural juice. Whey protein is a great low-fat, low-GI drink that can be found in health food stores and some supermarkets
ALTERNATIVE:
Small carton of low-fat fruit yogurt ½ cup

Lunch

Small carton of low-fat hummus
about ½ cup, served with 3 rye crispbreads and crudités of carrot, cucumber, celery, and cherry tomatoes

Snack

Handful of white grapes 2 oz

Dinner

Pork balls with tomato sauce and spaghetti
(see recipe, right)
ALTERNATIVE:
Spaghetti bolognese
made using 3 oz ground turkey or chicken per person, mixed with a 13 oz jar of ready-made, tomato pasta sauce. Serve with 3 oz, dry weight, of spaghetti per person

Going up

Today's rule is never to take the elevator or escalator. Climbing stairs gives you a workout. Each minute you climb burns 11 calories. Aim for 20–30 minutes of stair climbing today.

Calories burnt: 220–330

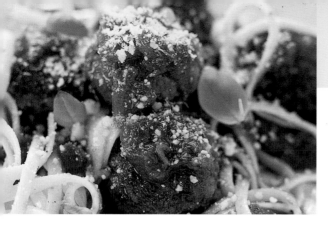

NUTRITION TIP

Pureed tomatoes are a great source of lycopene, a vital antioxidant which has been shown to reduce the risk of lung, prostate, and skin cancers.

Pork balls with tomato sauce and spaghetti

Preparation time 10 minutes **Cooking time** 20 minutes **Serves** 4

12 oz dried spaghetti
10 oz ground pork
1 onion, finely chopped
1 garlic clove, crushed
½ teaspoon paprika
2 teaspoons tomato paste
2½ cups pureed tomatoes
salt and pepper

• Cook the spaghetti in lightly salted boiling water for 12 minutes, or according to package instructions.

• Meanwhile, mix together the pork, onion, garlic, and paprika and season with salt and pepper. Shape the mixture into 12 balls.

• Place the meatballs on a broiler pan and cook under a preheated hot broiler for 6–7 minutes, turning occasionally, until browned and cooked through.

• Drain spaghetti, return it to the saucepan and stir in the tomato paste, pureed tomatoes and the meatballs. Season to taste with salt and pepper, heat through and serve.

kcal 486 (2041 kj) **protein** 27 g **carbohydrate** 78 g **fat** 9 g **GI** L

Did you know?

Eating a traditional high-carbohydrate diet is the equivalent of eating 2 cups of pure sugar a day. A low-GI diet produces dramatically less than this.

Day 3

By now you should be feeling some of the positive mental effects of the low-GI programme. One thing you should really notice is that pre- or post-meal mood swings have stopped, as you are not subjecting your body to sudden rises and falls in sugar levels that can make you grumpy and irritable.

Breakfast

Pumpkin seed and apricot muesli
(see recipe, right)
Glass of unsweetened grapefruit juice
⅔ cup

ALTERNATIVE:
Granola
½ cup of any unsweetened granola, topped with ⅔ cup skim or soy milk
½ grapefruit

Snack

½ mango
topped with ¼ cup low-fat cottage cheese

Lunch

Open tuna sandwich
made from 1 slice of multigrain, barley, or soy bread, topped with 3 oz of canned tuna in brine mixed with a little lemon juice and 1 teaspoon of low-fat mayonnaise, 1 sliced tomato, and a handful of alfalfa sprouts
Can or carton of lentil soup
13 oz

Snack

10 almonds
2 satsumas or kiwi fruit

Dinner

Broiled chicken breast
5 oz, served with ¼ cup of couscous (dry weight, cooked according to package instructions) and 6 oz of broiled vegetables—try a mix of eggplant, red bell pepper, zucchini and onion

Get dancing

Book a girls' night out and hit the local salsa, flamenco, or disco class. If you prefer to keep your moves to yourself, put on your favorite music and dance around the house for 20–30 minutes. Music is a great motivator for any exercise—studies show that a workout feels easier when it's done to music you enjoy.

Calories burnt: 100 for every 10 minutes

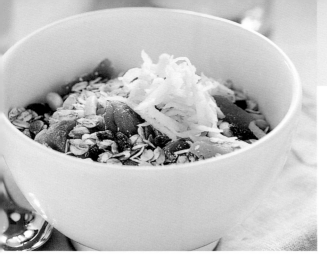

NUTRITION TIP

If you're not a morning person, make this muesli the night before. Carry out step 1 and put the mixture in the refrigerator overnight. In the morning, add the apples and milk. This will give a soft-textured muesli.

Pumpkin seed and apricot muesli

Preparation time 10 minutes   **Serves** 2

½ cup rolled jumbo oats

1 tablespoon golden raisins or raisins

1 tablespoon pumpkin or sunflower seeds

1 tablespoon chopped almonds

3 tablespoons ready-to-eat dried apricots, chopped

2 tablespoons orange or apple juice

2 small dessert apples, peeled and shredded

3 tablespoons skim or soy milk

• Place the oats, raisins, seeds, almonds, and apricots in a bowl with the fruit juice.

• Add the grated apples and stir to mix. Top with your chosen milk and serve.

kcal 340 (1428 kj)   **protein** 10 g   **carbohydrate** 39 g   **fat** 12 g   **GI** L

Motivation booster

Hunger on the low-GI plan is often psychological. If you feel hungry, as portion sizes look less than you're used to, use a smaller plate. It will look full, so you'll feel fuller.

Day 4

You are halfway through your first week and your insulin levels will be starting to level out. Your body will have started to burn fat for fuel—and you will have lost at least ½ lb. Don't get on the scales yet though—instead, just focus on the fact that every day from now means more weight lost.

Breakfast

Bowl of noodle-shaped bran cereal
1 cup, topped with ⅔ cup skim or soy milk and 1 sliced banana
Glass of unsweetened grapefruit juice
⅔ cup

Snack

Small carton of tzatziki
½ cup, served with 4 celery sticks

Lunch

Herby lentil salad with bacon
(see recipe, right)
ALTERNATIVE:
Quick lentil salad
Mix 2½ cups rinsed and drained canned lentils with 3 oz of lean ham, 3 chopped scallions, 1 tablespoon of chopped parsley, a squeeze of lemon juice, and season to taste

Snack

Blueberry smoothie
made from ⅔ cup soy milk, ½ cup soy yogurt and 4 oz blueberries

Dinner

Scallops with pasta
Pan-fry 8–10 bay scallops per person in a little lemon juice and oil from an oil spray. Serve with 2 oz of pasta spirals per person, on a bed of mixed salad leaves, sliced tomato, red bell pepper, and cucumber
ALTERNATIVE:
Shrimp with pasta
If you can't find scallops, use 5 oz shrimp per person, cooked in a little lemon juice and garlic

Circuit training

Do a little circuit training—this works all the muscles of your body and the variety stops you getting bored or too tired. A simple circuit would be 1 minute each of jogging on the spot, star jumps, skipping, stair climbing and sprinting between two points. Do the workout in your garden, the park, or even in the house and repeat as many times as you like.

Calories burnt: 50 per circuit

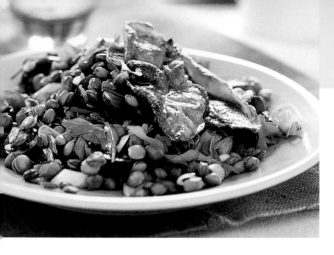

NUTRITION TIP

Today you have two recipes using an oil spray. Get a spray bottle from a kitchen shop and half fill with olive oil, then top up with water. Every time a recipe calls for oil to moisten a pan for frying, spritz with this to save calories.

Herby lentil salad with bacon

Preparation time 10 minutes   **Cooking time** 5 minutes   **Serves** 4

oil spray (see tip, above)

1 garlic clove, crushed

4 scallions, sliced

2 x 13 oz cans green lentils, drained and rinsed

2 tablespoons balsamic vinegar

3 tablespoons chopped herbs (such as parsley, oregano, or basil)

4 oz cherry tomatoes, halved

3 oz) Canadian bacon slices

• Spray a nonstick pan with oil, add the garlic and scallions and fry for 2 minutes.

• Stir in the lentils, vinegar, herbs, and tomatoes and set aside (or if you're taking this to work, put the salad in an airtight container until you want to eat it).

• Broil the bacon until crisp, place on top of the salad and serve. If you're eating at work, wrap the cooked, crisped bacon in paper towel, then foil. Add just before you eat.

kcal 313 (1314 kJ)   **protein** 24 g   **carbohydrate** 27 g   **fat** 12 g   **GI** L

Did you know?

We are only aware of 30 percent of the sugar that we eat—the other 70 percent is hidden in processed foods. Always read labels carefully and choose brands with no sugar, or those where it appears towards the end of the ingredients list.

Day 5

You should be appreciating the fill-up factor of this eating plan—and not experiencing hunger pangs or cravings you get on normal weight-loss diets. The only sign to show that you're on a diet is that your clothes are looser.

Breakfast

Omelet
made from 1 whole egg and 3 egg whites
Fill with ½ cup shredded low-fat cheddar cheese. Serve with 1 broiled tomato
Glass of any unsweetened fruit juice
⅔ cup

ALTERNATIVE:
Cold platter
1 oz lean ham, 1 oz cheese,
1 sliced tomato, 1 slice of dark rye bread with wholegrains (or multigrain, soy or barley bread)
Glass of any unsweetened orange or apple juice
⅔ cup

Snack

1 pear or apple
3 tablespoons of pumpkin seeds

Lunch

Tabbouleh salad
(see recipe, right), served with 4 oz sliced cooked chicken

Snack

2 rye crispbreads
spread with 2 oz low-fat pâté
White grapes 2 oz

Dinner

Cod in parsley sauce
Melt a teaspoon of butter in a pan with 2 tablespoons of white wine. Poach a 3 oz cod steak in the pan with a tablespoon of chopped parsley. Season and serve with ¼ cup quinoa or buckwheat, cooked according to package instructions, and unlimited carrots, broccoli, and kale

Mental workout

Give the hardcore exercise a rest today, and do some yoga instead. Not only will it help lengthen your muscles, it will also still your mind—good news, as stress increases levels of fat-storing hormones in the system.

Calories burnt: 150–600 per hour

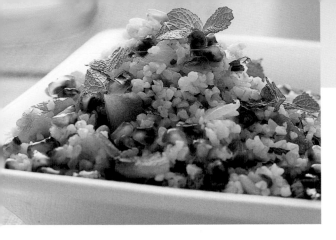

NUTRITION TIP
Rich in B vitamins, iron, phosphorus, and manganese, bulgar is one of the most nutritious of the grains. It also contains the heart-protecting vitamin E.

Tabbouleh salad

Preparation time 15 minutes, plus standing   **Serves** 4

1 cup bulgar wheat

1¼ cups boiling water

1 red onion, finely chopped

3 tomatoes, diced

½ cucumber, chopped

10 tablespoons chopped
   parsley

5 tablespoons chopped mint

Dressing

½ cup lemon juice

2 teaspoons olive oil

freshly ground black pepper

• Place the bulgar wheat in a bowl. Pour over the boiling water and let stand for 30 minutes, or according to package instructions, until the grains swell and soften.

• Drain the bulgar wheat and press to remove the excess moisture. Place in a salad bowl. Add the onion, tomatoes, cucumber, parsley, and mint. Toss to combine.

• Place all the dressing ingredients in a screw-top jar, replace the lid and shake well to combine. Pour over the salad and toss well.

kcal 193 (810 kj)   **protein** 5 g   **carbohydrate** 36 g   **fat** 3 g   **GI** L

Diet power-up

Green tea is a great low-GI beverage—but as well as this it has been shown to help increase the cells' response to insulin—and boost calorie burning. Four cups a day stokes the metabolic rate by around 4 percent, leading to an extra 65 calories a day burnt painlessly.

Day 6

If you started this diet on a Monday, this will be your first weekend day on the plan—don't let this throw you. You can still enjoy your weekend and stick to your diet—and if you do decide to go out for a meal, don't think you've automatically blown it. Just try to order within the low-GI rules and get back on the plan tomorrow.

Breakfast
Buckwheat pancakes (see recipe, right)
ALTERNATIVE:
1 boiled egg with 2 rye crispbreads topped with yeast extract
Serve with half a grapefruit and a smoothie made with ⅔ cup skim milk and 4 handfuls of blueberries, strawberries, or raspberries

Snack
1 slice of toast
Choose multigrain, barley, or soy bread and top with 1 tablespoon of peanut butter

Lunch
Bean salad
(see recipe, bottom right), topped with 4 oz canned tuna in spring water, 8 baby carrots and 5 cherry tomatoes

Snack
1 apple or orange

Dinner
Salmon steak
5 oz. Serve with 6 asparagus spears sprinkled with 3 tablespoons freshly grated Parmesan cheese then broiled until the cheese melts and the asparagus spears slightly char, and 4 oz of new potatoes and 3 oz of peas

Get into skating
Go in-line skating. If the weather's cold—or you don't own blades—try ice-skating instead. Both will tone your bottom, thighs, and stomach.
Calories burnt: 315 in 30 minutes

Motivation booster
Don't forget that nibbling while you are cooking can sabotage your diet by providing unwanted calories—chew sugar-free gum while you cook to prevent this.

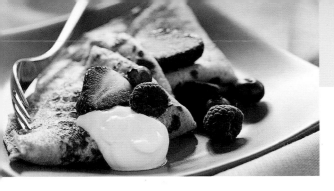

NUTRITION TIP
Buckwheat is a good source of lysine, an amino acid. Our body can't make it and relies on getting supplies from food. Lysine helps to absorb calcium.

Buckwheat pancakes

Preparation time 5 minutes, plus standing   **Cooking time** 25 minutes   **Serves** 4

½ cup whole wheat flour
½ cup buckwheat flour
1 egg
1¼ cups skim milk
8 teaspoons olive oil
fresh fruit and low-fat plain yogurt, to serve

• Sift the flours into a bowl and add the grains left in the sifter. Beat the egg and milk together, then add to the flour. Stir until a smooth batter forms. If the mixture is too thick, add a little milk. Let stand for 20 minutes, then stir.

• Put 1 teaspoon of oil in a nonstick skillet. When hot, add 2 tablespoons of pancake mixture and spread it over the pan. Cook for 2 minutes until the underside is lightly browned, turn and cook the other side for a minute or so.

• Keep the pancake warm in the oven while cooking the rest.

kcal 230 (966 kj)   **protein** 7 g   **carbohydrate** 13 g   **fat** 5 g   **GI** L

Bean salad

Preparation time 10 minutes   **Cooking time** 3 minutes   **Serves** 1

3 oz sliced green beans
¼ cup canned red kidney beans, rinsed and drained
2 tablespoons canned chickpeas, rinsed, drained
¼ onion, finely chopped
1 teaspoon chopped cilantro
1 teaspoon olive oil
salt and pepper

• Cook the green beans in lightly salted boiling water for 3 minutes, then drain and refresh under cold running water.

• Mix together all the ingredients in a bowl and serve.

kcal 161 (676 kj)   **protein** 7 g   **carbohydrate** 20 g   **fat** 6 g   **GI** L

Day 7

Halfway through, so today would be a good day to gauge your progress. Either step on the scales, or use your tape measure to see what you have lost and from where. Remember that losing weight isn't the only benefit you will have achieved by now: think about your improved energy levels and moods.

Breakfast
Cooked breakfast
2 slices of Canadian bacon trimmed of all fat, broiled mushroom, broiled tomato, 4 oz of canned baked beans and 1 slice of barley or multigrain toast

Snack
1 orange or 3 satsumas
Glass of skim or soy milk
²/₃ cup

Lunch
Roast lunch
5 oz roast chicken, beef, or pork (no skin, crackling, or other fat). Serve with 2 roast sweet potatoes, unlimited carrots, green beans, and Brussels sprouts, and 1 tablespoon of gravy

Snack
2 graham crackers
spread with a little fruit conserve

Dinner
Warm eggplant salad
(see recipe, right). Serve with a 5 oz sole or cod fillet, broiled or poached, and a large salad of mixed leaves topped with a little low-fat salad dressing, or lemon juice and black pepper

Enjoyable exercise

Exercise can be fun. Choose any of the following to burn 150 calories today.

- Play ten-pin bowling for 40 minutes
- Wash the car (by hand) for 37 minutes
- Play pool for 1 hour
- Mow the lawn for 23 minutes
- Walk the dog for 30 minutes
- Play catch for 20 minutes
- Window-shop for 1 hour
- Play table tennis or badminton for 25 minutes

Genius weight-loss plan

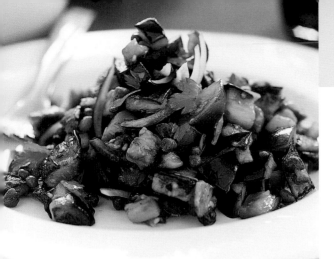

NUTRITION TIP

Eggplants are a good source of folic acid and contain lots of cancer-beating antioxidants. They tend to soak up oil, though, so be careful when cooking.

Warm eggplant salad

Preparation time 10 minutes, plus cooling   **Cooking time** 10 minutes   **Serves** 4

2 tablespoons olive oil

2 eggplants, cut into small cubes

1 red onion, finely sliced

2 tablespoons capers, roughly chopped

4 tomatoes, chopped

4 tablespoons chopped parsley

1 tablespoon balsamic vinegar

salt and pepper

• Heat the oil in a nonstick skillet (or use your oil spray to cut calories further). Add the eggplants and fry for 10 minutes until golden and softened.

• Add the onion, capers, tomatoes, parsley, and vinegar and stir to combine. Season lightly to taste. Remove from the heat and allow to cool for 10 minutes before serving.

kcal 99 (416 kj)   **protein** 3 g   **carbohydrate** 9 g   **fat** 6 g   **GI** L

Did you know?

Not getting enough sleep makes cells more resistant to insulin and may therefore promote fat storage. This is even more important when you realize that fatigue is one of the top three reasons why many of us reach for sugary or high-fat snacks. Try to get eight hours sleep a night.

Day 8

By now you will have noticed a definite change in your energy levels—you should be waking up feeling alert and not having mid-afternoon or early evening slumps. Use your new-found get-up-and-go to enjoy yourself—the more active you become, the better life is (and the more weight you lose).

Breakfast

Wake-up smoothie
made from 2 oz strawberries, 2 oz raspberries, ⅔ cup of orange juice and ¼ inch sliver of fresh gingerroot (peeled). Process in a blender until smooth

2 slices of toast
Choose multigrain, barley, or soy bread and top each with 1 teaspoon of peanut butter

Snack

Small carton of low-fat hummus
about ½ cup, with 2 carrots cut into crudités

Lunch

Cherry tomato and pasta salad
Cook 2 oz dried penne, cool and mix with 6 halved cherry tomatoes, ½ yellow bell pepper, sliced, ¼ cup of pine nuts, and 1½ tablespoons of grated Parmesan cheese. Add a squeeze of lemon juice, season to taste, and serve with watercress

Snack

Carton of low-fat fruit yogurt ½ cup

Dinner

Pan-fried lamb with spiced flageolet beans
(see recipe, right), served with 4 oz of broccoli and snow peas per person

ALTERNATIVE:

Grilled lean lamb chop
about 5 oz, served with 1 cup of canned lima beans, 100 g 4 oz of broccoli and snow peas and 1 tablespoon of gravy

Pushing harder

Go for a 30-minute walk, run, swim, or bicycle ride. Every 2 minutes, go as fast as you can for 30–60 seconds. Slow for 2 minutes, then do another fast spurt.

Calories burnt:
20 percent more than normal
- **170 for a walk**
- **260 for a swim**
- **360 for a run or bicycle ride**

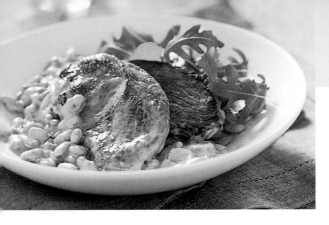

Pan-fried lamb with spiced flageolet beans

Preparation time 10 minutes, plus marinating   **Cooking time** 12 minutes   **Serves** 4

½ teaspoon ground cumin

½ teaspoon ground coriander

pinch of chili powder

1 tablespoon olive oil

4 lean lamb steaks

1 onion, sliced

1 garlic clove, crushed

4 tablespoons lemon juice

13 oz can flageolet beans, drained and rinsed

1 tablespoon chopped mint

2 tablespoons low-fat natural yogurt

• Mix together the cumin, coriander, chili, and half the oil in a non-metallic bowl. Add the lamb, coat it in the spices and set aside for 10 minutes.

• Heat the remaining oil in a nonstick pan, add the onion and garlic and fry for 3–4 minutes until softened.

• Add the lamb and the marinade and fry the steaks for 2–3 minutes on each side—or until cooked to your liking.

• Add the lemon juice, flageolet beans, mint, and natural yogurt and simmer for 1 minute until warmed through.

kcal 261 (1096 kj)   **protein** 26 g   **carbohydrate** 16 g   **fat** 12 g   **GI** L

Motivation booster

If you can't summon the energy to workout, take a sniff of peppermint oil, or eat a mint before starting. Exercisers run faster and feel stronger after inhaling the smell of mint.

Day 9

By now your clothes should be feeling slightly looser around the waist, hips or thighs—and if you've been exercising regularly you should also have started to notice some firming of your legs, bottom, and tummy muscles. Really focus on the gains you are making and remember that each day you carry on means more benefits to your body.

Breakfast
Scrambled eggs
made from 2 eggs, a splash of milk, and a dab of butter. Serve on 1 slice of multigrain, soy or barley toast

Snack
2 kiwi fruit or 2 handfuls of cherries

Lunch
Crab and avocado burrito
Spread 1 whole wheat tortilla wrap with a little salsa. Fill with 2 oz of crab meat (fresh or canned) and ½ avocado, sliced. Wrap up and serve with ¾ cup of canned red kidney beans, mixed with a little crushed garlic, chili powder, lemon juice, and olive oil

Snack
Protein shake (see page 46)

Dinner
Spicy lentil and tomato soup
(see recipe, right), served with a 4 oz chunk of multigrain, barley, or soy bread
ALTERNATIVE:
Carton of lentil, minestrone, or vegetable soup
13 oz, served with bread, as above

Going backward

To avoid boring gym workouts, try the treadmill backward. Holding the handrails, walk or run backwards for 5 minutes—it burns up to 32 percent more calories than going forward, as you take more steps.

Diet power-up

Are you drinking enough water? Being dehydrated not only gives you thirst cravings that many of us mistake for hunger, it also slows your metabolism.

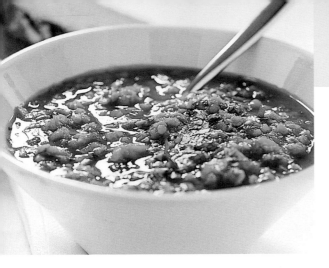

NUTRITION TIP

Soups are great diet foods as the combination of fluid and fiber fills you up. This one works well as it contains lentils, which are particularly filling, and metabolism-boosting chilies.

Spicy lentil and tomato soup

Preparation time 10–15 minutes   **Cooking time** 40–50 minutes   **Serves** 4

1 cup red lentils

1 tablespoon vegetable oil

1 large onion, finely chopped

1 garlic clove, finely chopped

1 celery stick, finely chopped

7 oz can chopped tomatoes, drained

½ small green chili, seeded and finely chopped (optional)

½ teaspoon paprika

½ teaspoon harissa paste

½ teaspoon ground cumin

2½ cups vegetable stock or water

salt and pepper

1 tablespoon chopped cilantro, to garnish

• Place the lentils in a bowl of water. Heat the oil in a large saucepan and gently fry the onion, garlic, and celery over a low heat until softened.

• Drain the lentils and add them to the vegetable pan with the tomatoes. Mix well. Add the chili, if using, paprika, harissa paste, cumin, and vegetable stock and season with salt and pepper. Cover the pan and simmer gently for about 30–40 minutes, until the lentils are soft, adding a little more vegetable stock or water if the soup gets too thick.

• Serve the soup immediately in warmed individual bowls topped with a little chopped cilantro.

kcal 288 (1210 kj)   **protein** 18 g   **carbohydrate** 28 g   **fat** 2 g   **GI** L

Day 10

Did you realize that so far following this diet plan you've eaten more fruit and vegetables than the average person eats in 10 weeks? Therefore, as well as all the health-boosting effects of a low-GI diet, you are also harnessing all the power of the nutrients and antioxidants found in fresh fruit and vegetables—no wonder you look and feel better already.

Breakfast
Bowl of porridge
(see page 44). Add 3 tablespoons of golden raisins and ½ apple, finely chopped, and mix well
Glass of unsweetened orange or grapefruit juice
⅔ cup

Snack
1 slice of multigrain, soy, or barley bread
topped with 1 oz tuna in spring water

Be a **water baby**

It doesn't matter what stroke you do, just aim to do 30 minutes of swimming today. You burn as many calories swimming a fast front crawl as you would running, but it feels easier as your body doesn't have to fight against gravity.

Calories burnt: 200–360

Lunch
Shrimp coleslaw
Mix 4 oz of peeled shrimps with 1 tablespoon reduced-fat mayonnaise and unlimited shredded white cabbage, carrot, and red onion. Serve with 1 small whole wheat pita bread

Snack
10 olives
5 almonds

Dinner
Ham steaks with creamy lentils
(see recipe, right), served with broccoli and green beans
ALTERNATIVE:
Broiled ham steak
5 oz, served with 1¼ cups of canned lentils tossed with a squeeze of lemon juice and some chopped herbs, and unlimited green vegetables

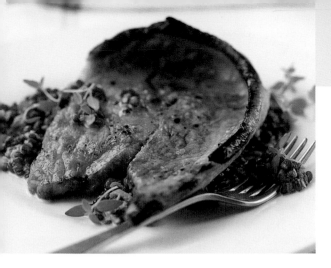

Ham steaks with creamy lentils

Preparation time 8 minutes   **Cooking time** 25–30 minutes   **Serves** 4

½ cup Puy lentils
¼ cup butter
2 shallots
1 garlic clove, chopped
2 thyme sprigs, crushed
1 teaspoon cumin seeds
4 teaspoons Dijon mustard
2 teaspoons honey
4 ham steaks, 5 oz each
½ cup hard cider
⅓ cup light cream
salt and pepper

• Place the lentils in a pan and cover with cold water. Bring to a boil and cook for 20 minutes.

• Meanwhile, melt the butter in a skillet and fry the shallots, garlic, thyme, and cumin seeds, stirring frequently, for 10 minutes until the shallots are soft and golden.

• Blend the mustard and honey and season to taste with salt and pepper. Brush the mixture over the ham steaks and broil for 3 minutes on each side until golden and cooked through. Keep warm.

• Drain the lentils and add them to the shallot mixture. Pour in the cider, bring to a boil and cook until reduced to about 4 tablespoons. Stir in the cream, heat through and season to taste with salt and pepper. Serve with the ham steaks, garnished with thyme leaves.

kcal 420 (1764 kj)   **protein** 22 g   **carbohydrate** 35 g   **fat** 21 g   **GI** L

Day 11

You may be noticing more beneficial effects of the GI diet by now. Those prone to skin breakouts may have found them less severe. And by avoiding the sugars that cause inflammation, your skin may look smoother and younger. On top of this, the fact that you are getting protein from a variety of sources, and plenty of calcium, means your hair and nails are benefiting too.

Breakfast

Cottage cheese and fruit
½ cup of low-fat cottage cheese mixed with 1 sliced banana, 1 sliced pear, a handful of berries, and ½ mango. Serve with 1 slice of fruit bread, toasted

Snack

2 rye crispbreads
topped with 1 teaspoon of hummus and 1 sliced tomato

Lunch

Chicken caesar salad
4 oz of broiled chicken and unlimited iceberg lettuce mixed with 1 tablespoon of low-fat caesar salad dressing, topped with 1½ tablespoons grated Parmesan
Can or carton of minestrone, tomato, or lentil soup
13 oz

Snack
2 satsumas

Dinner

Teriyaki salmon on noodles
(see recipe, right), served with unlimited steamed bok choy

ALTERNATIVE:
Broiled salmon steak
6 oz, served with 2 oz of dry egg noodles, cooked according to package instructions, unlimited bok choy, and 1 teaspoon of sweet chili sauce

Learn something new

Try a different exercise class: great calorie-burners are Step, Spinning or Kickboxing classes, while Pump, Pilates or Sculpt classes are good body-toners. If you can't get out, hire an exercise video: salsa, martial arts, Tae Bo, or general aerobics tapes need no special equipment.

Calories burnt:
400–600 per hour for calorie burners
150–300 for toners

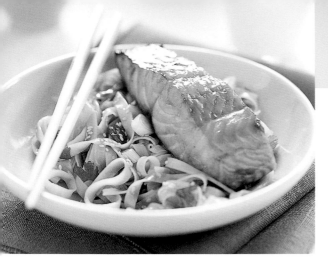

Teriyaki salmon on noodles

Preparation time 10 minutes, plus marinating **Cooking time** 12 minutes **Serves** 4

4 skinless salmon fillets, about
  4 oz each

2 tablespoons soy sauce

1 tablespoon dry sherry

2 tablespoons brown sugar

2 garlic cloves, crushed

1 teaspoon grated fresh
  gingerroot

1 tablespoon sesame oil

2 tablespoons water

2 tablespoons sesame seeds

2 scallions, chopped

8 oz dried rice noodles, cooked
  according to package
  instructions

3 tablespoons chopped cilantro
  leaves

• Place the salmon on a foil-lined broiler pan. Mix together
the soy sauce, sherry, sugar, garlic, ginger, half of the oil, and
the water. Brush half the marinade over the salmon and set
aside for 10 minutes.

• Cook the salmon under a preheated hot broiler for
5–6 minutes, turning it halfway through the cooking time
and brushing with a little more of the marinade.

• Meanwhile, heat the remaining oil in a saucepan, add the
sesame seeds and scallions and fry for 1 minute. Add the
noodles and any remaining marinade to the saucepan and
heat through. Stir in the cilantro. Serve the salmon on a bed
of noodles.

kcal 504 (2117 kj) **protein** 30 g **carbohydrate** 50 g **fat** 20 g **GI** L

Day 12

You're on the home stretch and by now your body should really start to be regaining control of its insulin levels. As a result, it's time for a treat. Whichever treat you choose this afternoon, make sure you really enjoy it.

Breakfast

Walnut and banana sunrise smoothie
(see recipe, right)

Bowl of cereal
½ cup noodle-shaped bran cereal, topped with ⅔ cup of skim milk and 2 oz of berries

ALTERNATIVE:

Glass of unsweetened orange, grapefruit, or cranberry juice
⅔ cup

Bowl of cereal
½ cup noodle-shaped bran cereal topped with ⅔ cup of skim milk, 2 oz of berries, and 2 tablespoons of chopped walnuts

Snack

Small carton of tzatziki
½ cup, served with 2 carrots cut into crudités

Lunch

Open sandwich
made from 1 slice of multigrain, barley, or soy bread, spread with a little mustard and topped with 2 oz of ham, and 2 oz of cooked sliced chicken or turkey. Add sliced tomatoes, cucumber, and lettuce.

Bean salad
(see recipe, page 55) 4 oz

Snack

Sweet treat
choose from: 1 oz dark or milk chocolate, 2 scoops of any low-fat ice cream or frozen yogurt, or 2 chocolate cookies

Dinner

Steak or sole
5 oz sirloin steak or sole fillet, broiled and served with 3 oz of roasted or mashed sweet potatoes and 3 oz of peas

Do some **weights**

Go to the gym and use the weights—if you don't know how, ask an instructor to show you. Weight training not only tones your body, it also helps build muscle.

Calories burnt: 150 in 30 minutes

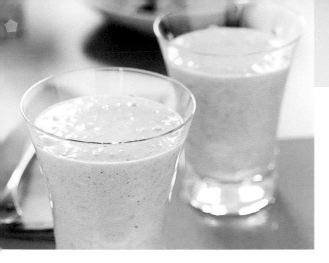

Walnut and banana sunrise smoothie

Preparation time 10 minutes   **Serves** 2

1 orange, segmented

1 banana

²/₃ cup soy or skim milk

½ cup soy or plain yogurt

¼ cup walnut pieces

1 teaspoon honey

• Place all the ingredients in a food processor or blender and blend until smooth and frothy. Pour into two glasses and serve.

kcal 265 (1113 kj) (skim milk), 273 (1146 kj) (soy milk)   **protein** 10 g
carbohydrate 35 g (skim milk), 30 g (soy milk)   **fat** 11 g (skim milk), 13 g (soy milk)   **GI** L

Motivation booster

If your diets are destroyed by comfort eating when you're bored or upset, simply tell yourself that the food won't cheer you up as much as a hot bath or a chat to friends. When researchers at Case Western University in Chicago asked volunteers to do this, their snack consumption fell.

Day 13

You could be surprised that this morning starts with a full cooked breakfast —but everything in this meal is a low-GI food, meaning you can eat it and still lose weight. Use it to power up another active weekend.

Breakfast
Cooked breakfast
1 boiled or poached egg, 1 slice of lean Canadian bacon or one low-fat sausage broiled, 4 oz of canned baked beans and 3 broiled mushrooms
Glass of unsweetened orange juice
²/₃ cup

Snack
4 oz strawberries

Lunch
Falafel salad
6 grilled falafel balls, served with a large salad of arugula, bean sprouts, tomato, green bell pepper and ½ avocado

Snack
Cheese and grapes
2 oz Edam or low-fat cheddar and 4 oz red grapes

Dinner
Griddled chicken with pearl barley
(see recipe, right)
ALTERNATIVE:
Broiled chicken with pasta
5 oz broiled chicken breast, served with 2 oz of dried pasta spirals or ¼ cup of dried lentils, cooked according to package instructions, and a large mixed salad

Get adventurous

If there's an indoor (or outdoor) ski slope near you, strap on some skis. If there's a rock climbing wall, then go and climb it. Or try your first horse ride. While you are learning something new, it won't feel like exercise.

Calories burnt: 400–600 per hour

Diet power-up

Fidget—tapping your fingers, swinging a leg, running up and down all burn calories, to the extent that fidgeters burn 800 calories more a day than those who sit still.

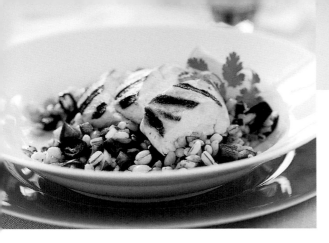

Griddled chicken with pearl barley

Preparation time 50 minutes   **Cooking time** 10 minutes   **Serves** 4

4 boneless, skinless chicken
  breasts

1 tablespoon olive oil

½ cup pearl barley, cooked
according to package
instructions

1 red onion, finely chopped

1 red chili, finely chopped

4 tablespoons chopped cilantro
  leaves

grated zest and juice of 2 limes

1 red bell pepper, cored,
  seeded, and finely chopped

salt and pepper

cilantro leaves and lime
  wedges to garnish

• Brush each chicken piece with a little oil. Heat a griddle
pan until hot and cook the chicken for 4–5 minutes on each
side until golden and cooked through. Cut each breast into
4 slices.

• Stir the remaining oil into the barley and add the onion,
chili, cilantro, lime zest and juice, and red bell pepper. Season
to taste with salt and pepper and stir to combine.

• Serve the barley topped with the chicken, garnished with
parsley and lime wedges.

kcal 360 (1512 kj)   **protein** 40 g   **carbohydrate** 30 g   **fat** 10 g   **GI** L

Day 14

This is the end of your organized plan—get on the scales, or grab a tape measure and see how you have done. But just because the plan is over, it doesn't mean your weight loss efforts have to be—you can either repeat the program as many times as it takes to get to your desired weight, or use the low-GI rules to create your own plan.

Breakfast

Buckwheat pancakes
(see recipe, page 55), served with 1 sliced banana and 1 teaspoon of maple syrup
Glass of soya or skim milk
⅔ cup

Snack

⅔ **tablespoon of almonds**
2 oz raspberries

Lunch

Salmon salad
4 oz of canned salmon or tuna in spring water, drained and served with a large green salad and 3 oz of boiled new potatoes

Snack

Carton of low-fat yogurt
½ cup

Dinner

Vegetable curry
(see recipe, right), served with 2 tablespoons of dried basmati rice and ¼ cup of dried lentils, cooked according to package instructions, plus a serving of spinach sprinkled with a little lemon juice and nutmeg
ALTERNATIVE:
Ready-made vegetable curry
Choose one with under 300 kcal (1260 kj).
Serve with rice, lentils, and spinach

Get competitive

Try playing your partner or a friend at a one-on-one sport like tennis, squash, or badminton. It's great fun and provides a good work-out.

Calories burnt: 300 per 30-minute game

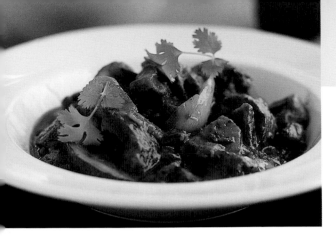

NUTRITIONAL TIP

Coconut milk contains saturated fat so you shouldn't eat it every day, but it does give a great flavor to curries. Just choose reduced-fat versions—and remember, some studies show coconut milk can boost the immune system.

Vegetable curry

Preparation time 10 minutes   **Cooking time** 25 minutes   **Serves** 4

1 tablespoon olive oil

1 onion, chopped

1 garlic clove, crushed

2 tablespoons medium curry paste

3 lb prepared vegetables (such as zucchini, sweet peppers, squash, mushrooms, and green beans)

7 oz can chopped tomatoes

13 oz can reduced-fat coconut milk

2 tablespoons chopped cilantro leaves

• Heat the oil in a large saucepan (or use your oil spray as before), add the onion and garlic and fry for 2 minutes. Stir in the curry paste and fry for 1 minute more.

• Add the vegetables and fry for 2–3 minutes, stirring occasionally, then add the tomatoes and coconut milk. Stir well, bring to a boil then lower the heat and simmer for 12–15 minutes or until all the vegetables are cooked. Stir in the cilantro and serve.

kcal 268 (1125 kj)   **protein** 6 g   **carbohydrate** 35 g   **fat** 11 g   **GI** L

Did you know?

Sunlight helps the brain create serotonin and may help reduce the amount of carbohydrates you crave. If you're missing any foods, try and get outside today to boost your health.

GI charts

This is the section for those who need to adapt the calorie count for their diet. Here you will find calorie counts for every food included in the GI weight-loss diets.

However, this is also the section for anyone who wants to take low-GI eating into their daily life. Listed here is the GI rating for over 300 day-to-day foods—everything from alfalfa sprouts to yogurt. Using these charts, you can make GI eating the permanent way to good health, increased energy, a slimmer figure—and possibly even a longer life.

Using the charts

Foods are listed in alphabetical order, as well as under section headings, such as Beans and legumes, to make comparisons easy. You'll find the foods are marked clearly as high, medium, or low GI. Underneath each listing you'll see how many calories (kcal) or kilojoules (kj) there are in 1 oz of the food (or ½ cup) if it's a liquid).

Items marked with O are pure protein foods that have a negligible effect on blood sugar and while not officially measured, their glycemic index is assumed to be low. Note that processing (for example, beefburgers rather than beef steak), adding bread crumbs, butter, or sauces, can change the GI of these foods. All measurements (unless a processed product is noted) are for the pure product, such as fresh chicken breast or fresh fish fillet.

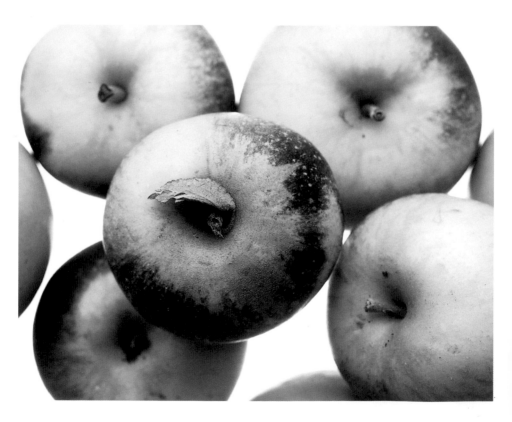

A

	LOW	MED	HIGH
Alfalfa 7 kcal (29 kj)	●		
Almonds 172 kcal (722 kj)	●		
Anchovies 76 kcal (320 kj)	○		
Angler fish 18 kcal (76 kj)	○		
Apple 13 kcal (55 kj)	●		
Apple juice 43 kcal (180 kj)	●		
Apricots 8 kcal (34 kj)		●	
Apricots (canned) 18 kcal (76 kj)		●	
Apricots (dried) 53 kcal (223 kj)	●		
Artichoke 13 kcal (55 kj)	●		
Asparagus 25 kcal (105 kj)	●		
Avocado 54 kcal (227 kj)	●		

B

	LOW	MED	HIGH
Bacon (Canadian) 53 kcal (222 kj)	○		
Bagel 68 kcal (286 kj)			●
Baguette 77 kcal (323 kj)			●
Baked beans 23 kcal (97 kj)	●		
Baked potato 21 kcal (88 kj)			●
Banana 26 kcal (110 kj)		●	
Barley bread (no grains) 48 kcal (202 kj)		●	

	LOW	MED	HIGH
Barley bread (with grains) 44 kcal (184 kj)	●		
Basmati rice (dried) 97 kcal (407 kj)		●	
Basmati rice (cooked) 36 kcal (151 kj)		●	
Beans and legumes			
Baked beans 23 kcal (97 kj)	●		
Black-eyed beans (dried) 77 kcal (323 kj)	●		
Black-eyed beans (canned) 32 kcal (134 kj)	●		
Chana dhal 30 kcal (125 kj)	●		
Chickpeas (dried) 91 kcal (382 kj)	●		
Chickpeas (canned) 33 kcal (139 kj)	●		
Fava beans (fresh) 17 kcal (71 kj)			●
Fava beans (canned) 25 kcal (105 kj)			●
Flageolet beans 25 kcal (105 kj)	●		
Kidney beans (dried) 76 kcal (320 kj)	●		
Kidney beans (canned) 29 kcal (121 kj)	●		
Lentils (dried) 90 kcal (378 kj)	●		
Lentils (canned) 30 kcal (126 kj)	●		

	GI VALUE		
	LOW	MED	HIGH
Lima beans (dried) 83 kcal (349 kj)	●		
Lima beans (canned) 22 kcal (92 kj)	●		
Navy beans (dried) 82 kcal (344 kj)	●		
Navy beans (cooked) 27 kcal (113 kj)	●		
Soy beans (dried) 106 kcal (445 kj)	●		
Soy beans (cooked) 40 kcal (168 kj)	●		
Split peas (dried) 94 kcal (395 kj)	●		
Split peas (cooked) 36 kcal (151 kj)	●		
Bean sprouts 9 kcal (38 kj)	●		
Beef (lean cuts) 50 kcal (210 kj)	○		
Beef ground (lean) 50 kcal (210 kj)	○		
Beer 32 kcal (134 kj)			●
Beet 10 kcal (42 kj)		●	
Black-eyed beans (canned) 32 kcal (134 kj)	●		
Black-eyed beans (dried) 77 kcal (323 kj)	●		
Blackberries 7 kcal (29 kj)	●		
Blueberries 8 kcal (34 kj)	●		

	GI VALUE		
	LOW	MED	HIGH
Boiled potatoes 21 kcal (88 kj)	●		
Bran cereal (flakes) 90 kcal (378 kj)			●
Bran cereal (noodle shaped) 76 kcal (320 kj)	●		
Bran cereal (with fruit) 90 kcal (378 kj)		●	
Brazil nuts 198 kcal (831 kj)	●		
Bread and cakes Bagel 68 kcal (286 kj)			●
Baguette 77 kcal (323 kj)			●
Barley bread (no grains) 48 kcal (202 kj)		●	
Barley bread (with grain) 44 kcal (184 kj)	●		
Bread stuffing (made up) 35 kcal (147 kj)			●
Brown bread 62 kcal (260 kj)		●	
Croissant 80 kcal (336 kj)		●	
Crumpet 45 kcal (189 kj)		●	
Doughnut 99 kcal (416 kj)			●
Fruit bread 85 kcal (357 kj)	●		
Gluten-free bread 100 kcal (420 kj)			●
Muffin (plain) 90 kcal (378 kj)		●	
Muffin (fruit) 100 kcal (420 kj)		●	
Multigrain bread 61 kcal (256 kj)	●		

Food	LOW	MED	HIGH
Pancakes 73 kcal (307 kj)		●	
Pastry 130 kcal (546 kj)		●	
Pita bread (white) 62 kcal (260 kj)		●	
Pita bread (brown) 61 kcal (256 kj)		●	
Rye/pumpernickel bread (with grains) 46 kcal (193 kj)	●		
Rye/pumpernickel (no grains) 90 kcal (378 kj)		●	
Scones (plain) 75 kcal (315 kj)			●
Stoneground bread 60 kcal (252 kj)		●	
Sourdough bread 63 kcal (264 kj)		●	
Soy bread 64 kcal (269 kj)	●		
Sponge cake 81 kcal (340 kj)	●		
Tortilla wraps (white) 81 kcal (340 kj)		●	
Tortilla wraps (wheat) 79 kcal (331 kj)	●		
Waffles 110 kcal (462 kj)			●
White bread 62 kcal (260 kj)			●
White bread (added fiber) 61 kcal (256 kj)		●	
Whole wheat bread 61 kcal (256 kj)		●	

Breakfast cereals

Food	LOW	MED	HIGH
Bran cereal (flakes) 90 kcal (378 kj)			●
Bran cereal (with fruit) 90 kcal (378 kj)		●	
Bran cereal (noodle shaped) 76 kcal (320 kj)	●		
Cornflakes 105 kcal (441 kj)			●
Granola 105 kcal (441 kj)		●	
Granola (low sugar) 101 kcal (424 kj)		●	
Honey-coated cereals 106 kcal (445 kj)			●
Porridge (instant, dried) 111 kcal (466 kj)		●	
Porridge oats (dried) 105 kcal (441 kj)	●		
Rice cereal 93 kcal (390 kj)			●
Wheat cereal 95 kcal (399 kj)		●	
Broccoli 9 kcal (38 kj)	●		
Brown bread 62 kcal (260 kj)		●	
Brown rice (dried) 100 kcal (420 kj)		●	
Brown rice (cooked) 40 kcal (168 kj)		●	
Brussels sprouts 12 kcal (50 kj)	●		
Buckwheat (dried) 102 kcal (428 kj)	●		
Bulgar wheat (dried) 104 kcal (437 kj)	●		
Butter 206 kcal (865 kj)	●		

C

	LOW	MED	HIGH
Cabbage 8 kcal (37 kj)	●		
Camembert 85 kcal (357 kj)	○		
Cantaloupe melon 5 kcal (21 kj)		●	
Capers 8 kcal (37 kj)	●		
Carrots 10 kcal (42 kj)	●		
Carrot juice 27 kcal (113 kj)	●		
Cashew nuts 176 kcal (740 kj)	●		
Cauliflower 10 kcal (42 kj)	●		
Celery 2 kcal (8 kj)	●		
Chana dhal 30 kcal (125 kj)	●		
Cheddar 116 kcal (487 kj)	○		
Cheddar (half fat) 75 kcal (315 kj)	○		
Cheeses			
Camembert 85 kcal (357 kj)	○		
Cheddar 116 kcal (487 kj)	○		
Cheddar (half fat) 75 kcal (315 kj)	○		
Cottage cheese 27 kcal (113 kj)	○		
Cottage cheese (half fat) 22 kcal (92 kj)	○		
Cream cheese 80 kcal (336 kj)	○		
Cream cheese (half fat) 50 kcal (210 kj)	○		

	LOW	MED	HIGH
Edam 95 kcal (399 kj)	○		
Edam (half fat) 70 kcal (294 kj)	○		
Feta 75 kcal (315 kj)	○		
Mozzarella 88 kcal (369 kj)	○		
Parmesan 108 kcal (453 kj)	○		
Ricotta 53 kcal (222 kj)	○		
Stilton 101 kcal (424 kj)	○		
Cherries 11 kcal (46 kj)	●		
Chicken (meat only) 32 kcal (134 kj)	○		
Chicken (meat and skin) 37 kcal (155 kj)	○		
Chicken nuggets 43 kcal (180 kj)	●		
Chickpeas (dried) 91 kcal (382 kj)	●		
Chickpeas (canned) 33 kcal (139 kj)	●		
Chips 140 kcal (588 kj)			●
Chocolate (milk) 153 kcal (643 kj)	●		
Chocolate (dark) 128 kcal (535 kj)	●		
Chocolate (white) 150 kcal (630 kj)	●		
Chocolate (low-fat, milk) 81 kcal (340 kj)	●		
Chocolate-covered peanuts 128 kcal (537 kj)	●		

	GI VALUE		
	LOW	MED	HIGH
Chocolate spread 154 kcal (647 kj)	●		
Cod fillet 21 kcal (88 kj)	○		
Cola 43 kcal (181 kj)		●	
Condensed milk 17 kcal (71 kj)		●	
Cookies and crackers			
Graham crackers 150 kcal (630 kj)		●	
Melba toast 99 kcal (416 kj)			●
Oatcakes 123 kcal (516 kj)		●	
Rice cakes 92 kcal (386 kj)			●
Rye crispbreads 88 kcal (370 kj)		●	
Shortbread 120 kcal (504 kj)		●	
Soda crackers 124 kcal (520 kj)		●	
Tea cookies 112 kcal (470 kj)		●	
Corn 19 kcal (80 kj)		●	
Cornflakes 105 kcal (441 kj)			●
Corn chips 57 kcal (249 kj)		●	
Corn kernals 35kcal (147 kj)		●	
Cottage cheese 27 kcal (113 kj)	○		
Cottage cheese (half fat) 22 kcal (92 kj)	○		
Couscous (dried) 03 kcal (433 kj)		●	
Couscous (cooked) 48 kcal (201 kj)		●	

	GI VALUE		
	LOW	MED	HIGH
Crab meat 37 kcal (155 kj)	○		
Cranberry juice 51 kcal (214 kj)		●	
Cream cheese 80 kcal (336 kj)	○		
Cream cheese (half fat) 50 kcal (210 kj)	○		
Croissant 80 kcal (336 kj)		●	
Crumpet 45 kcal (189 kj)		●	
Cucumber 3 kcal (13 kj)	●		
Custard 1 oz powder made with skim milk) 22 kcal (92 kj)	●		
Custard 1 oz powder made with whole milk) 33 kcal (139 kj)	●		

D

	GI VALUE		
	LOW	MED	HIGH
Dairy products			
Chocolate milk (low-fat) 81 kcal (340 kj)	●		
Condensed milk 17 kcal (71 kj)		●	
Ice cream (low fat) 42 kcal (176 kj)	●		
Ice cream (full fat) 70 kcal (294 kj)		●	
Lowfat milk 45 kcal (189 kj)	●		
Skim milk 34 kcal (142 kj)	●		
Sour cream 188 kcal (789 kj)	●		

	GI VALUE		
	LOW	MED	HIGH
Whole milk 65 kcal (273 kj)	●		
Yogurt 23 kcal (97 kj)	●		
Yogurt (low fat) 15 kcal (63 kj)	●		
Dates (fresh) 31 kcal (130 kj)			●
Dates (dried) 77 kcal (323 kj)			●
Doughnuts 99 kcal (416 kj)			●
Drinks			
Apple juice 43 kcal (180 kj)	●		
Beer 32 kcal (134 kj)			●
Carrot juice 27 kcal (113 kj)	●		
Chocolate milk (low-fat) 81 kcal (340 kj)	●		
Cola 43 kcal (181 kj)		●	
Cranberry juice 51 kcal (214 kj)		●	
Glucose drinks 76 kcal (320 kj)			●
Grapefruit juice 35 kcal (147 kj)	●		
Orange juice 40 kcal (168 kj)	●		
Orange soda 43 kcal (181 kj)		●	
Pineapple juice 45 kcal (189 kj)	●		
Sports drinks 28 kcal (118 kj)	●		
Tomato juice 15 kcal (63 kj)	●		

	GI VALUE		
	LOW	MED	HIGH
Water 0 kcal (0 kj)	●		
Wine (white) 66 kcal (277 kj)		●	
Wine (red) 68 kcal (285 kj)		●	
Duck (meat only) 53 kcal (223 kj)	○		
Duck (meat and skin) 94 kcal (395 kj)	○		
E			
Edam 95 kcal (399 kj)	○		
Edam (half fat) 70 kcal (294 kj)	○		
Eggplant 18 kcal (75 kj)	●		
Eggs (medium) 80 kcal (336 kj)	○		
Egg noodles 109 kcal (458 kj)	●		
Egg white 15 kcal (63 kj)	○		
F			
Falafel 37 kcal (155 kj)	●		
Fava beans (fresh) 17 kcal (71 kj) 74 g			●
Fava beans (canned) 25 kcal (105 kj)			●
Feta 75 kcal (315 kj)	○		
Fettucine (white, dried) 103 kcal (432 kj)	●		

	GI VALUE		
	LOW	MED	HIGH
Fettucine (white, cooked) 33 kcal (138 kj)	●		
Figs (fresh) 12 kcal (50 kj)		●	
Figs (dried) 65 kcal (273 kj)		●	
Fish and shellfish			
Anchovies 76 kcal (320 kj)	○		
Angler fish 18 kcal (76 kj)	○		
Cod fillet 21 kcal (88 kj)	○		
Crab meat 37 kcal (155 kj)	○		
Fish fingers 44 kcal (185 kj)	●		
Flounder 27 kcal (113 kj)	○		
Haddock 20 kcal (84 kj)	○		
Halibut 29 kcal (122 kj)	○		
Kipper 46 kcal (193 kj)	○		
Lobster 33 kcal (139 kj)	○		
Mackerel 62 kcal (260 kj)	○		
Mussels (shelled) 25 kcal (105 kj)	○		
Mussels (with shells) 9 kcal (38 kj)	○		
Pilchards 40 kcal (168 kj)	○		
Salmon (fresh) 50 kcal (210 kj)	○		

	GI VALUE		
	LOW	MED	HIGH
Salmon (canned) 44 kcal (185 kj)	○		
Sardines (fresh) 46 kcal (193 kj)	○		
Sardines (canned in oil) 61 kcal (256 kj)	○		
Scallops 21 kcal (88 kj)	○		
Shrimp (peeled) 30 kcal (126 kj)	○		
Sole fillet 26 kcal (109 kj)	○		
Swordfish 31 kcal (130 kj)	○		
Trout fillet 38 kcal (160 kj)	○		
Tuna (fresh) 40 kcal (168 kj)	○		
Tuna (canned in spring water) 28 kcal (118 kj)	○		
Tuna (canned in oil) 53 kcal (223 kj)	○		
Fish fingers 44 kcal (185 kj)	●		
Flounder 27 kcal (113 kj)	○		
French fries (thick cut) 54 kcal (227 kj)			●
French fries (thin cut) 80 kcal (336 kj)			●
Fruits			
Apple 13 kcal (55 kj)	●		
Apricots 8 kcal (34 kj)		●	

	GI VALUE		
	LOW	MED	HIGH
Apricots (canned) 18 kcal (76 kj)		●	
Apricots (dried) 53 kcal (223 kj)	●		
Avocado 54 kcal (227 kj)	●		
Banana 26 kcal (110 kj)		●	
Blackberries 7 kcal (29 kj)	●		
Blueberries 8 kcal (34 kj)	●		
Cantaloupe melon 5 kcal (21 kj)		●	
Cherries 11 kcal (46 kj)	●		
Figs (fresh) 12 kcal (50 kj)		●	
Figs (dried) 65 kcal (273 kj)		●	
Fruit cocktail (canned in juice) 8 kcal (34 kj)		●	
Fruit cocktail (canned in syrup) 16 kcal (68 kj)		●	
Golden raisins 79 kcal (332 kj)		●	
Grapefruit 9 kcal (38 kj)	●		
Grapes (white) 16 kcal (67 kj)	●		
Grapes (red) 16 kcal (67 kj)		●	
Kiwi fruit 12 kcal (50 kj)	●		
Lemons 4 kcal (17 kj)	●		
Limes 2 kcal (8 kj)	●		

	GI VALUE		
	LOW	MED	HIGH
Mandarin 11 kcal (46 kj)	●		
Mango 16 kcal (67 kj)		●	
Olives 34 kcal (143 kj)	●		
Oranges 7 kcal (30 kj)	●		
Papaya 10 kcal (42 kj)		●	
Peaches 8 kcal (34 kj)	●		
Peaches (canned in juice) 11 kcal (46 kj)	●		
Peaches (canned in syrup) 16 kcal (67 kj)		●	
Pears 12 kcal (50 kj)	●		
Pears (canned in juice) 9 kcal (38 kj)	●		
Pears (canned in syrup) 14 kcal (59 kj)		●	
Pineapple 12 kcal (50 kj)		●	
Pineapple (canned in juice) 13 kcal (55 kj)		●	
Pineapple (canned in syrup) 18 kcal (76 kj)		●	
Plums 10 kcal (420 kj)	●		
Prunes 38 kcal (160 kj)	●		
Raisins 78 kcal (328 kj)		●	
Raspberries 7 kcal (29 kj)	●		
Satsumas 11 kcal (46 kj)	●		

	GI VALUE		
	LOW	MED	HIGH
Strawberries 8 kcal (34 kj)	●		
Watermelon (with skin) 5 kcal (21 kj)			●
Watermelon (skinned) 9 kcal (38 kj)			●
Tomatoes 5 kcal (21 kj)	●		
Tomatoes (canned) 5 kcal (21 kj)	●		
Fruit bread 85 kcal (357 kj)	●		
Fruit cocktail (canned in juice) 8 kcal (34 kj)		●	
Fruit cocktail (canned in syrup) 16 kcal (68 kj)		●	

G

	LOW	MED	HIGH
Gluten-free bread 100 kcal (420 kj)			●
Gluten-free pasta 100 kcal (420 kj)		●	
Glucose drinks 76 kcal (320 kj)			●
Golden raisins 79 kcal (332 kj)		●	
Goose 89 kcal (374 kj)	○		
Graham crackers 150 kcal (630 kj)		●	
Granola 105 kcal (441 kj)		●	
Granola (low sugar) 101 kcal (424 kj)		●	
Granola bars 101 kcal (424 kj)		●	
Grapefruit 9 kcal (38 kj)	●		

	GI VALUE		
	LOW	MED	HIGH
Grapefruit juice 35 kcal (147 kj)	●		
Grapes (white) 16 kcal (67 kj)	●		
Grapes (red) 16 kcal (67 kj)		●	
Guacamole 53 kcal (222 kj)	●		

H

	LOW	MED	HIGH
Haddock 20 kcal (84 kj)	○		
Halibut 29 kcal (122 kj)	○		
Ham (reduced fat) 32 kcal (134 kj)	○		
Ham steak (fat removed) 47 kcal (197 kj)	○		
Hamburger roll 80 kcal (336 kj)		●	
Hard candy 100 kcal (420 kj)			●
Honey 85 kcal (357 kj)		●	
Honey-coated cereal 106 kcal (445 kj)			●
Hummus 85 kcal (357 kj)	●		

I

	LOW	MED	HIGH
Ice cream (low fat) 42 kcal (176 kj)	●		
Ice cream (full fat) 70 kcal (294 kj)		●	
Instant mash (dried) 90 kcal (378 kj)			●
Instant mash (reconstituted) 15 kcal (63 kj)			●

	LOW	MED	HIGH
Instant noodles 85 kcal (357 kj)	●		
J			
Jasmine rice 98 kcal (412 kj)			●
Jelly 75 kcal (315 kj)	●		
Jelly beans 92 kcal (386 kj)			●
K			
Kidney beans (dried) 76 kcal (320 kj)	●		
Kidney beans (canned) 29 kcal (121 kj)	●		
Kippers 46 kcal (193 kj)	○		
Kiwi fruit 12 kcal (50 kj)	●		
L			
Lamb chop (with fat) 88 kcal (370 kj)	○		
Lamb (lean) 57 kcal (240 kj)	○		
Leeks 6 kcal (25 kj)	●		
Lemons 4 kcal (17 kj)	●		
Lentils (dried) 90 kcal (378 kj)	●		
Lentils (canned) 30 kcal (126 kj)	●		
Lentil soup 23 kcal (97 kj)	●		
Lettuce 4 kcal (17 kj)	●		

	LOW	MED	HIGH
Lima beans (dried) 83 kcal (349 kj)	●		
Lima beans (canned) 22 kcal (92 kj)	●		
Limes 2 kcal (8 kj)	●		
Linguine (dried) 103 kcal (432 kj)	●		
Lobster 33 kcal (139 kj)	○		
Lowfat milk 45 kcal (189 kj)	●		
Low-fat spread 106 kcal (445 kj)	●		
M			
Mackerel 62 kcal (260 kj)	○		
Mandarin 11 kcal (46 kj)	●		
Margarine 204 kcal (856 kj)	●		
Mashed potato (real) 21 kcal (88 kj)			●
Mashed potato (instant) 15 kcal (63 kj)			●
Macaroni 103 kcal (432 kj)	●		
Mango 16 kcal (67 kj)		●	
Marmalade 72 kcal (30 kj)	●		
Meats			
Bacon (Canadian) 53 kcal (222 kj)	○		
Beef (lean cuts) 50 kcal (210 kj)	○		

Food	GI VALUE LOW	MED	HIGH
Beef (lean ground) 50 kcal (210 kj)	○		
Ham (reduced fat) 32 kcal (134 kj)	○		
Ham steak (fat removed) 47 kcal (197 kj)	○		
Lamb chop (with fat) 88 kcal (370 kj)	○		
Lamb (lean) 57 kcal (240 kj)	○		
Pork (meat only) 59 kcal (248 kj)	○		
Pork chop (lean) 53 kcal (223 kj)	○		
Pork chop (with fat) 73 kcal (307 kj)	○		
Sausages 80 kcal (336 kj)	●		
Sirloin steak 54 kcal (227 kj)	○		
Veal 65 kcal (273 kj)	○		
Venison 30 kcal (126 kj)	○		
Melba toast 99 kcal (416 kj)			●
Millet 104 kcal (437 kj)			●
Milks			
Chocolate milk (low-fat) 81 kcal (340 kj)	●		
Condensed milk 17 kcal (71 kj)		●	
Lowfat 45 kcal (189 kj)	●		
Skim 34 kcal (142 kj)	●		

Food	GI VALUE LOW	MED	HIGH
Soy milk 43 kcal (180 kj)	●		
Whole milk 65 kcal (273 kj)	●		
Mozzarella 88 kcal (369 kj)	○		
Muffin (plain) 90 kcal (378 kj)		●	
Muffin (fruit) 100 kcal (420 kj)		●	
Multigrain bread 61 kcal (256 kj)	●		
Mussels (shelled) 25 kcal (105 kj)	○		
Mussels (with shells) 9 kcal (38 kj)	○		

N

Food	GI VALUE LOW	MED	HIGH
Navy beans (dried) 82 kcal (344 kj)	●		
Navy beans (cooked) 27 kcal (113 kj)	●		
Nut oils 899 kcal (3775 kj)	●		

O

Food	GI VALUE LOW	MED	HIGH
Oatcakes 123 kcal (516 kj)			●
Oils and fats			
Butter 206 kcal (865 kj)	●		
Low-fat spread 106 kcal (445 kj)	●		
Margarine 204 kcal (856 kj)	●		
Nut oils 899 kcal (3775 kj)	●		
Olive oil 899 kcal (3775 kj)	●		

Food	LOW	MED	HIGH
Vegetable oil 900 kcal (3780 kj)	●		
Olives 34 kcal (143 kj)	●		
Olive oil 899 kcal (3775 kj)	●		
Onions 10 kcal (420 kj)	●		
Oranges 7 kcal (30 kj)	●		
Orange juice 40 kcal (168 kj)	●		
Orange soda 43 kcal (181 kj)		●	

P

Food	LOW	MED	HIGH
Pancakes 73 kcal (307 kj)		●	
Papaya 10 kcal (420 kj)		●	
Parmesan 108 kcal (453 kj)	○		
Parsnips 18 kcal (76 kj)			●
Pasta, rice and grains			
Basmati rice (dried) 97 kcal (407 kj)		●	
Basmati rice (cooked) 36 kcal (151 kj)		●	
Brown rice (dried) 100 kcal (420 kj)		●	
Brown rice (cooked) 40 kcal (168 kj)		●	
Buckwheat (dried) 102 kcal (428 kj)	●		
Bulgar wheat (dried) 104 kcal (437 kj)	●		

Food	LOW	MED	HIGH
Couscous (dried) 103 kcal (433 kj)		●	
Couscous (cooked) 48 kcal (201 kj)		●	
Egg noodles 109 kcal (458 kj)	●		
Fettucine (white, dried) 103 kcal (432 kj)	●		
Fettucine (white, cooked) 33 kcal (138 kj)	●		
Gluten-free pasta 100 kcal (420 kj)			●
Instant noodles 85 kcal (357 kj)	●		
Jasmine rice 98 kcal (412 kj)			●
Linguine (dried) 103 kcal (432 kj)	●		
Macaroni 103 kcal (432 kj)	●		
Millet 104 kcal (437 kj)			●
Pearl barley 101 kcal (424 kj)	●		
Quinoa 87 kcal (365 kj)	●		
Ravioli (meat, dried) 78 kcal (328 kj)	●		
Ravioli (meat, cooked) 46 kcal (193 kj)	●		
Ravioli (cheese, dried) 95 kcal (399 kj)	●		
Ravioli (cheese, cooked) 57 kcal (238 kj)	●		

	GI VALUE		
	LOW	MED	HIGH
Risotto rice 101 kcal (424 kj)		●	
Spaghetti (white, dried) 103 kcal (432 kj)	●		
Spaghetti (white, cooked) 33 kcal (138 kj)	●		
Spaghetti (brown, dried) 96 kcal (403 kj)	●		
Spaghetti (brown, cooked) 32 kcal (134 kj)	●		
Tortellini (meat, dried) 78 kcal (328 kj)	●		
Tortellini (meat, cooked) 46 kcal (193 kj)	●		
Tortellini (cheese, dried) 95 kcal (399 kj)	●		
Tortellini (cheese, cooked) 57 kcal (238 kj)	●		
Udon noodles 86 kcal (361 kj)		●	
Vermicelli (dried) 103 kcal (433 kj)	●		
Vermicelli (cooked) 34 kcal (143 kj)	●		
White rice (dried) 108 kcal (453 kj)		●	
White rice (cooked) 39 kcal (164 kj)		●	
White rice (fast cook, dried) 108 kcal (453 kj)			●
White rice (fast cook, cooked) 39 kcal (164 kj)			●

	GI VALUE		
	LOW	MED	HIGH
Wild rice (dried) 104 kcal (437 kj)		●	
Wild rice (cooked) 50 kcal (210 kj)		●	
Pastry 130 kcal (546 kj)		●	
Pâté 85 kcal (357 kj)	●		
Pâté (low fat) 50 kcal (210 kj)	●		
Peaches 8 kcal (34 kj)	●		
Peaches (canned in syrup) 16 kcal (67 kj)			●
Peanuts 160 kcal (672 kj)	●		
Peanuts (chocolate-covered) 128 kcal (537 kj)	●		
Peanut butter 150 kcal (630 kj)	●		
Pearl barley 101 kcal (424 kj)	●		
Pears 12 kcal (50 kj)	●		
Pears (canned in juice) 9 kcal (38 kj)	●		
Peas 24 kcal (100 kj)	●		
Pilchards 40 kcal (168 kj)	○		
Pineapple 12 kcal (50 kj)			●
Pineapple (canned in juice) 13 kcal (55 kj)			●
Pineapple (canned in syrup) 18 kcal (76 kj)			●

	GI VALUE		
	LOW	MED	HIGH
Pineapple juice 45 kcal (189 kj)	●		
Pinenuts 193 kcal (810 kj)	●		
Pita bread (white) 80 kcal (336 kj)		●	
Pita bread (brown) 80 kcal (336 kj)		●	
Pizza (meat, thin crust) 62 kcal (260 kj)	●		
Pizza (vegetarian, thin crust) 58 kcal (244 kj)	●		
Plums 10 kcal (420 kj)	●		
Popcorn 100 kcal (420kg)			●
Pork (meat only) 59 kcal (248 kj)	○		
Pork chop (lean) 53 kcal (223 kj)	○		
Pork chop (with fat) 73 kcal (307 kj)	○		
Porridge (instant, dried) 111 kcal (466 kj)		●	
Porridge oats (dried) 105 kcal (441 kj)	●		
Potatoes			
Baked 21 kcal (88 kj)			●
Chips 140 kcal (588 kj)		●	
French fries (thick cut) 54 kcal (227 kj)			●
French fries (thin cut) 80 kcal (336 kj)			●
Mashed (real) 21 kcal (88 kj)			●

	GI VALUE		
	LOW	MED	HIGH
Mashed (instant) 15 kcal (63 kj)			●
New 20 kcal (84 kj)	●		
Sweet potatoes 25 kcal (105 kj)		●	
Yam 33 kcal (139 kj)		●	
Poultry and game			
Chicken (meat only) 32 kcal (134 kj)	○		
Chicken (meat and skin) 37 kcal (155 kj)	○		
Chicken nuggets 43 kcal (180 kj)	●		
Duck (meat only) 53 kcal (223 kj)	○		
Duck (meat and skin) 94 kcal (395 kj)	○		
Goose 89 kcal (374 kj)	○		
Turkey (meat only) 45 kcal (189 kj)	○		
Turkey (meat and skin) 52 kcal (218 kj)	○		
Pretzels 91 kcal (382 kj)			●
Pumpkin 4 kcal (17 kj)			●
Pumpkin seeds 159 kcal (667 kj)	●		

Q

Quinoa 87 kcal (365 kj)	●		
Quorn™ 24 kcal (100 kj)	●		

R

	LOW	MED	HIGH
Raisins 78 kcal (328 kj)		●	
Raspberries 7 kcal (29 kj)	●		
Ravioli (cheese, dried) 95 kcal (399 kj)	●		
Ravioli (cheese, cooked) 57 kcal (238 kj)	●		
Ravioli (meat, dried) 78 kcal (328 kj)	●		
Ravioli (meat, cooked) 46 kcal (193 kj)	●		
Rice			
Basmati (dried) 97 kcal (407 kj)		●	
Basmati (cooked) 36 kcal (151 kj)		●	
Brown rice (dried) 100 kcal (420 kj)		●	
Brown rice (cooked) 40 kcal (168 kj)		●	
Jasmine rice 98 kcal (412 kj)			●
Risotto rice 101 kcal (424 kj)		●	
White (dried) 108 kcal (453 kj)		●	
White (cooked) 39 kcal (164 kj)		●	
White (fast cook, dried) 108 kcal (453 kj)			●
White (fast cook, cooked)			●

	LOW	MED	HIGH
39 kcal (164 kj)			
Wild rice (dried) 104 kcal (437 kj)		●	
Wild rice (cooked) 50 kcal (210 kj)		●	
Rice cakes 92 kcal (386 kj)			●
Rice cereal (plain) 100 kcal (420 kj)			●
Rice cereal (chocolate) 108 kcal (453 kj)			●
Rice noodles (dried) 102 kcal (428 kj)		●	
Rice noodles (cooked) 35 kcal (147 kj)		●	
Ricotta 53 kcal (222 kj)	○		
Risotto rice 101 kcal (424 kj)		●	
Rice cereals 93 kcal (390 kj)			●
Rutabaga 7 kcal (29 kj)			●
Rye bread 46 kcal (193 kj)		●	
Rye crispbreads 88 kcal (370 kj)		●	

S

	LOW	MED	HIGH
Salmon (fresh) 50 kcal (210 kj)	○		
Salmon (canned) 44 kcal (185 kj)	○		
Salsa 13 kcal (55 kj)	●		

	GI VALUE		
	LOW	MED	HIGH
Sardines (fresh) 46 kcal (193 kj)	○		
Sardines (canned in oil) 61 kcal (256 kj)	○		
Satsumas 11 kcal (46 kj)	●		
Sausages 80 kcal (336 kj)	●		
Scallops 21 kcal (88 kj)	○		
Scones (plain) 75 kcal (315 kj)			●
Shortbread 120 kcal (504 kj		●	
Shrimp (peeled) 30 kcal (126 kj)	○		
Sirloin steak 54 kcal (227 kj)	○		
Skim milk 34 kcal (142 kj)	●		
Snacks (savory)			
Almonds 172 kcal (722 kj)	●		
Brazil nuts 198 kcal (831 kj)	●		
Cashew nuts 176 kcal (740 kj)	●		
Chips (potato) 140 kcal (588 kj)		●	
Corn chips 57 kcal (249 kj)		●	
Peanuts 160 kcal (672 kj)	●		
Popcorn 100 kcal (420kg			●
Pretzels 91 kcal (382 kj)			●
Rice cakes 92 kcal (386 kj)			●
Walnuts 192 kcal (806 kj)	●		

	GI VALUE		
	LOW	MED	HIGH
Snacks (sweet)			
Chewy fruit sweets 105 kcal (441 kj)			●
Chocolate (milk) 153 kcal (643 kj)	●		
Chocolate (dark) 128 kcal (535 kj)	●		
Chocolate (white) 150 kcal (630 kj)	●		
Chocolate-covered peanuts 128 kcal (537 kj)	●		
Doughnuts 99 kcal (416 kj)			●
Graham cookies 150 kcal (630 kj)		●	
Granola bars 101 kcal (424 kj)		●	
Hard candy 100 kcal (420 kj)			●
Ice cream (low fat) 42 kcal (176 kj)	●		
Ice cream (full fat) 70 kcal (294 kj)		●	
Jelly beans 92 kcal (386 kj)			●
Muffin (plain) 90 kcal (378 kj)		●	
Muffin (fruit) 100 kcal (420 kj)		●	
Shortbread 120 kcal (504 kj)		●	
Sponge cake 81 kcal (340 kj)	●		
Tea cookies 112 kcal (470 kj)		●	
Yogurt 23 kcal (97 kj)	●		

	GI VALUE		
	LOW	MED	HIGH
Yogurt (low fat) 15 kcal (63 kj)	●		
Snow peas 9 kcal (37 kj)	●		
Soda crackers 80 kcal (336 kj)		●	
Sole fillet 26 kcal (109 kj)	○		
Sour cream 188 kcal (789 kj)	●		
Sourdough bread 63 kcal (264 kj)		●	
Soybeans (dried) 106 kcal (445 kj)	●		
Soybeans (cooked) 40 kcal (168 kj)	●		
Soy bread 64 kcal (269 kj)	●		
Soy milk 43 kcal (180 kj)	●		
Soy mince (granules) 74 kcal (310 kj)	●		
Spaghetti (white, dried) 103 kcal (432 kj)	●		
Spaghetti (white, cooked) 33 kcal (138 kj)	●		
Spaghetti (brown, dried) 96 kcal (403 kj)	●		
Spaghetti (brown, cooked) 32 kcal (134 kj)	●		
Spinach 7 kcal (29 kj)	●		
Split peas (dried) 94 kcal (395 kj)	●		

	GI VALUE		
	LOW	MED	HIGH
Split peas (cooked) 36 kcal (151 kj)	●		
Spreads and dips			
Chocolate spread 154 kcal (647 kj)	●		
Guacamole 53 kcal (222 kj)	●		
Honey 85 kcal (357 kj)		●	
Hummus 85 kcal (357 kj)	●		
Jelly 75 kcal (315 kj)	●		
Marmalade 72 kcal (30 kj)	●		
Peanut butter 150 kcal (630 kj)	●		
Salsa 13 kcal (55 kj)	●		
Sponge cake 81 kcal (340 kj)	●		
Sports drinks 28 kcal (118 kj)			●
Strawberries 8 kcal (34 kj)	●		
Stilton 101 kcal (424 kj)	○		
Stuffing (bread, made up) 35 kcal (147 kj)			●
Sweet peppers 5 kcal (21 kj)	●		
Sweet potatoes 25 kcal (105 kj)		●	
Swordfish 31 kcal (130 kj)	○		

T

	GI VALUE		
	LOW	MED	HIGH
Taco shells 120 kcal (504 kj)		●	
Tea cookies 112 kcal (470 kj)		●	

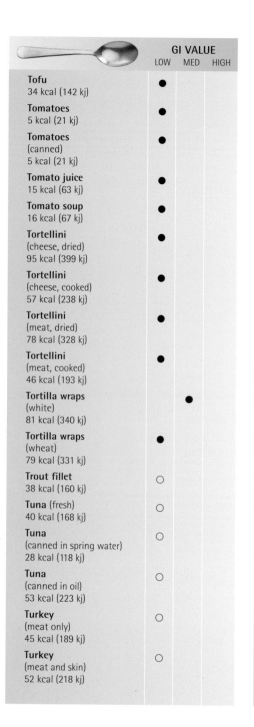

	GI VALUE		
	LOW	MED	HIGH
Tofu 34 kcal (142 kj)	●		
Tomatoes 5 kcal (21 kj)	●		
Tomatoes (canned) 5 kcal (21 kj)	●		
Tomato juice 15 kcal (63 kj)	●		
Tomato soup 16 kcal (67 kj)	●		
Tortellini (cheese, dried) 95 kcal (399 kj)	●		
Tortellini (cheese, cooked) 57 kcal (238 kj)	●		
Tortellini (meat, dried) 78 kcal (328 kj)	●		
Tortellini (meat, cooked) 46 kcal (193 kj)	●		
Tortilla wraps (white) 81 kcal (340 kj)		●	
Tortilla wraps (wheat) 79 kcal (331 kj)	●		
Trout fillet 38 kcal (160 kj)	○		
Tuna (fresh) 40 kcal (168 kj)	○		
Tuna (canned in spring water) 28 kcal (118 kj)	○		
Tuna (canned in oil) 53 kcal (223 kj)	○		
Turkey (meat only) 45 kcal (189 kj)	○		
Turkey (meat and skin) 52 kcal (218 kj)	○		

	GI VALUE		
	LOW	MED	HIGH
U			
Udon noodles 86 kcal (361 kj)		●	
V			
Veal 65 kcal (273 kj)	○		
Vegetables			
Alfalfa 7 kcal (29 kj)	●		
Artichoke 13 kcal (55 kj)	●		
Asparagus 25 kcal (105 kj)	●		
Bean sprouts 9 kcal (38 kj)	●		
Beet 10 kcal (42 kj)			●
Broccoli 9 kcal (38 kj)	●		
Brussels sprouts 12 kcal (50 kj)	●		
Cabbage 8 kcal (37 kj)	●		
Capers 8 kcal (37 kj)	●		
Carrots 10 kcal (42 kj)	●		
Cauliflower 10 kcal (42 kj)	●		
Celery 2 kcal (8 kj)	●		
Corncob 19 kcal (80 kj)		●	
Corn kernals 35 kcal (147 kj)		●	
Cucumber 3 kcal (13 kj)	●		
Eggplant 18 kcal (75 kj)	●		
Leeks 6 kcal (25 kj)	●		

	GI VALUE		
---	LOW	MED	HIGH
Lettuce 4 kcal (17 kj)	●		
Onions 10 kcal (420 kj)	●		
Parsnips 18 kcal (76 kj)			●
Peas 24 kcal (100 kj)	●		
Pumpkin 4 kcal (17 kj)			●
Rutabaga 7 kcal (29 kj)			●
Snow peas 9 kcal (37 kj)	●		
Spinach 7 kcal (29 kj)	●		
Sweet peppers 5 kcal (21 kj)	●		
Tomatoes 5 kcal (21 kj)	●		
Tomatoes (canned) 5 kcal (21 kj)	●		
Watercress 6 kcal (25 kj)	●		
Zucchini 5 kcal (21 kj)	●		
Vegetable oil 900 kcal (3780 kj)	●		
Venison 30 kcal (126 kj)	○		
Vermicelli (dried) 103 kcal (433 kj)	●		
Vermicelli (cooked) 34 kcal (143 kj)	●		

W

	LOW	MED	HIGH
Watercress 6 kcal (25 kj)	●		
Watermelon (with skin) 5 kcal (21 kj)			●
Watermelon (skinless) 9 kcal (38 kj)			●
Waffles 110 kcal (462 kj)			●

	GI VALUE		
---	LOW	MED	HIGH
Walnuts 192 kcal (806 kj)	●		
Wheat cereal 95 kcal (399 kj)		●	
Whey protein 4 kcal (17 kj)	○		
White bread 62 kcal (260 kj)			●
White bread (added fiber) 61 kcal (256 kj)		●	
White rice (dried) 108 kcal (453 kj)		●	
White rice (cooked) 39 kcal (164 kj)		●	
White rice (fast cook, dried) 108 kcal (453 kj)			●
White rice (fast cook, cooked) 39 kcal (164 kj)			●
Whole milk 65 kcal (273 kj)	●		
Whole wheat bread 61 kcal (256 kj)		●	
Wild rice (dried) 104 kcal (437 kj)		●	
Wild rice (cooked) 50 kcal (210 kj)		●	
Wine (white) 66 kcal (277 kj)		●	
Wine (red) 68 kcal (285 kj)		●	

Y

	LOW	MED	HIGH
Yam 33 kcal (139 kj)		●	
Yogurt 23 kcal (97 kj)	●		
Yogurt (low fat) 15 kcal (63 kj)	●		

Z

	LOW	MED	HIGH
Zucchini 5 kcal (21 kj)	●		

Index

Acknowledgments

Executive Editor	Nicky Hill
Editor	Jessica Cowie
Executive Art Editor	Rozelle Bentheim
Designer	Ginny Zeal
Senior Production Controller	Martin Croshaw
Special Photography	Ian O'Leary and Lis Parsons
Food Stylists	Beth Heald and David Morgan